I Choose Everything

Embracing Life in the Face of Terminal Illness

Jozanne Moss
Michael Wenham

16
EasyRead Large

RHYW

Copyright Page from the Original Book

Published by Monarch Books
an imprint of
Lion Hudson plc
Wilkinson House, Jordan Hill Road, Oxford OX2 8DR, England
Tel: +44 (0)1865 302750 Fax: +44 (0)1865 302757
Email: monarch@lionhudson.com
www.lionhudson.com

ISBN 978 0 85721 012 8

British Library Cataloguing Data
A catalogue record for this book is available from the British Library.

TABLE OF CONTENTS

"I often argue for the consistency and coherence of the Christian worldview. As compelling as my arguments may be, they are a poor substitute for the power of the living testimony of someone like Jozanne Moss."

– **ANDREL IMMELMAN,** CHRISTIAN APOLOGIST, SOUTH AFRICA

"In a society which is deeply afraid of death, this is a powerful witness to the Christian vision, not only of death, but of the meaning of everything. This is the fruit of an intensely lived experience."

– **THE VERY REVD DOMINIC MILROY,** OSB, OF AMPLEFORTH ABBEY

"We have seen Jozanne outwardly wasting away – but alongside we have also seen how she has been inwardly renewed ... God has used Jozanne in ways that are nothing short of remarkable. Her testimony of God's grace has touched the lives of many."

– **DR ERROL WAGNER,** SOUTH AFRICA

Dedication

Jozanne...

To the ones I love the most: my dear husband, Dave, and my brave and courageous children. Luke and Nicole, you make me extremely proud to be your mother. God has loved me through you and I am blessed. I love you always.

Michael...

To my brothers, Gordon, David and Peter, and my younger sister, Louise Halling, all of whom I love dearly, and in memory of two inspirational men who have completed this road before me, Tim Berner and John Walliker.

Acknowledgments

Jozanne...

This book would not have been possible without the hard work and dedication of my co-author, and now friend, Michael Wenham. I wrote down and shared my experiences with friends and family, but Michael worked tirelessly to put a book together. I am eternally grateful to you, Michael. Thank you for your vision.

In this book the story of my journey with MND is told. In it I mention many of the wonderful people who helped and supported us along the way, but there is one person who stands out above them all. Without my care-giver and friend, Idith Matolla, or Idie, as I fondly call her, I would not have been able to live this life. God chose her to walk alongside me. She was like my shadow and a part of me; what I couldn't do for myself anymore, she did for me, with the greatest love and respect. She was always there for me and for my family and I love her dearly. Thank you, Idie.

Lastly, but most importantly, thanks be to God for His grace and faithfulness. From the beginning I knew that God had a plan and a purpose with my illness. And look what He has done! Great is Thy faithfulness.

Michael...

My first acknowledgment must be to my co-author, Jozanne, and her husband, Dave. Although we have never met, God has given us a deep friendship, which has inspired and challenged me. One of the treats I have in store is meeting them and Luke and Nicole in a better country even than our present homes, one day.

Once again I have to thank my amazing wife, Jane, and all my family who continue to support and show me what love means, concealing what it costs.

Jozanne and I would like to thank Archbishop Desmond Tutu for agreeing to the Foreword. The claims of a South African mother and an English Anglican priest seemed rather a small call on his busy schedule, and we simply felt humbled and honoured when he said yes to our request.

There are many people whom I have met on my journey since publishing *My Donkeybody.* They are too many to mention but some of them appear in my parts of this book. In one way or another they have inspired, and challenged, me. One name I must mention, however, because without him this book would not exist, and that is Peter Saunders (General Secretary of the Christian Medical Fellowship). He introduced Jozanne to me in June 2009 – and the rest is this story!

Lastly, I am grateful to Tony Collins and Jenny Ward of Monarch Books for putting faith in another book and seeing it through to speedy publication. They are aware of the significance of that.

AMDG (To the greater glory of God)

Foreword

Every person is special to God. God loves each of us as if we were the only person on earth. And so when a Christian is afflicted by a terminal illness, she may naturally wonder, "Where are you, God, in this?" In this book, Jozanne and Michael ask just that question, because they both have the same degenerative disease. They are an odd couple! Jozanne is a teacher and mother; she lives in George in South Africa. Michael is an Anglican priest, who lives near Oxford in England. Now they are both facing death. Of course we all face death. But these two people know they are on death row. You could call this book "Dead men talking"! Because they have never been able to meet, they corresponded entirely by email, and this is the outcome of their correspondence.

I expected the book to be depressing, downbeat. But no! Not at all. It is honest. Both authors obviously have struggled with the way the disease removed their freedom, little by little, muscle by muscle. For each of them it has attacked their faith and spiritual life. Jozanne's diary in particular lets us see, in painful intimacy, the grievous prospect of losing everything and everyone she holds dear. And yet, everything *isn't* lost. That's the wonderful certainty that God gives his children. We're all part of his plan. We are all part of his family. St Paul says, "God chose us in Christ to be God's children before the foundation of the world." We didn't have to do anything. It was given freely and our worth is infinite. We aren't an afterthought. Isn't that beautiful? We aren't an accident. Some of us might look like accidents. But no, no one is an accident. Isn't it incredible?

None of God's sons and daughters is ordinary. Each of us is unique and loved just as we are. We are loved with an everlasting love, a love that will not let us go, by a God who did not spare his only Son. So this is a story of two ordinary Christians in extraordinary circumstances. I am sure that you will be moved and inspired by their testimony. This book was written in order to encourage other people who are in the shadow of death and in the desert of loneliness. It says, "You are not alone, whatever it feels like – because Christ has been there already, and he *is* there now." Amen!

Archbishop Emeritus Desmond Tutu
Cape Town

CHAPTER 1

Unanswered questions

One day Leonie, thinking no doubt that she was too big to play with dolls, brought us a basket filled with clothes, pretty pieces of stuff, and other trifles on which her doll was laid: "Here, dears," she said, "choose whatever you like." Celine looked at it, and took a woollen ball. After thinking about it for a minute, I put out my hand saying: "I choose everything," and I carried off both doll and basket without more ado.

THÉRÈSE OF LISIEUX[1]

In less than twenty years, Thérèse Martin had acute and agonizing tuberculosis. She suffered terribly, coughing blood from her lungs, experiencing breathlessness and suffocation. Eventually, her vital functions began to fail. No painkillers, such as morphine, were administered to relieve the agony. She died on 30 September 1897 in a convent in Northern France. She was only twenty-four. When her sister, Agnes, who was a nun, visiting her a week before her death, re-

---

1 The Story of a Soul, Chapter 1, trans. Thomas Taylor, Project Gutenberg Ebook, 2009.

marked, "What a terrible sickness and how much you suffered!", she replied, "Yes! What a grace it is to have faith! If I had not any faith, I would have committed suicide without an instant's hesitation." (Last Conversation, 22.9.6)

This is not a book about Thérèse of Lisieux, as she quite soon became known. But it *is* about choosing, and living, and dying. And it *is* about faith and the difference faith makes when you are facing illness, especially "incurable" illness. Particularly, it is about *choice.* It is often thought, or implied, that the world is divided into those who are "pro-life" and those who are "pro-choice". My observation is that this is a false antithesis. Thérèse Martin went on to write: "This childish incident was a forecast, so to speak, of my whole life ... then also, as in the days of my childhood, I cried out: 'My God, I choose everything, I will not be a saint by halves, I am not afraid of suffering for Thee, I only fear one thing, and that is to do my own will. Accept the offering of my will, for I choose all that Thou willest.'"[2] This is not a passive acceptance of whatever life throws at us; it is a positive choice to embrace the whole of life, whether we like it or not. It is a position of faith – for many, faith in God, but for many others faith in the value of life itself.

I have Primary Lateral Sclerosis, a relatively slow form of Motor Neurone Disease, about which I have

---

2 Thérèse of Lisieux, ibid.

written in *My Donkeybody – living with a body that no longer obeys you.*[3] (Motor Neurone Disease is also known as Lou Gehrig's Disease or Amyotrophic Lateral Sclerosis, but will be referred to as Motor Neurone Disease or MND here.) There, I primarily tried to paint a picture of what it's like to be diagnosed with a terminal condition and to live with the diagnosis. I wanted to get across the way the reality crept up on me, to the point where there was no doubting that the consultant's verdict was right: I had a fatal illness. And I wanted to get across the relentless progress (if you can call it progress) of the disease and its invasion of my body, emotions, and my whole existence. So I told my story. I told it for myself, of course, but I mainly told it for anyone who cared to read it, especially those facing the multitude of "terminal" degenerative conditions, and for the carers of those with these diseases. I was writing for people with faith or with no religious convictions, but I did not attempt to conceal my own faith.

However, for a Christian, of course, and indeed for anyone who is vaguely thoughtful, illnesses such as mine raise some profound questions which could not be avoided. So, in a few chapters of *My Donkeybody,* I have addressed them in a somewhat summary fashion. They were questions to do with the use of stem cells in research and treatment, assisted suicide, miraculous healing, and the consolation of an afterlife.

---

3 Monarch Books, Oxford, 2008.

But there were some big unanswered issues I was aware of by-passing. One was the question "Why?", "Why is this happening to me?", or, more fundamentally, "Why does a good God, if there is one, allow all this pain in his world?" Another was, "How does a Christian steer his or her way through the experience of suffering?"

I am not sure whether this book is going to provide theological (or, as a friend recently wryly observed, what this usually means: theoretical) answers. Since beginning this journey of illness, I have met several fellow-travellers and from them I have gained wonderful insights. One of them I have met only via the Internet. She is Jozanne Moss, who lives in George, near Cape Town in South Africa. We were "introduced" by Dr Peter Saunders in June 2009. We both have Motor Neurone Disease, but Jozanne's is of a more aggressive form than mine. That, and our shared faith, forged an immediate bond between us. Jozannne, who has two young children, seems to me someone who has chosen everything with inspiring faith. This book is largely inspired by our correspondence, of which the greater part was hers, and forms the chapters here entitled "Jozanne's Story".

We hope that this is not seen as a book about our particular condition. We hope that you read it as two twenty-first-century Christians struggling with the age-old questions raised by sickness and faith. It could equally have been written by those experiencing the panoply of other "incurable" diseases. God has just chosen to bring us together with the same illness and the same goal: to encourage and inspire others with the life God has purposed for us all.

Of course, if one looks in the pages of the Bible, there too one meets people of faith wrestling with the human condition. And, as the beginning of this chapter reminds us, saints throughout the ages have walked similar and harder roads.

This book is addressed specifically to those saints' successors. Not in the sense of "a bundle of bones which fools adore when life is o'er",[4] as Newman's chorus of demons mocked, but all those who have known "amazing grace". In other words, it is for Christians of all sorts, all ages, and all complexions, and perhaps in particular for those for whom the words of the old carol hold an aching resonance:

O ye beneath life's crushing load,
Whose forms are bending low,
Who toil along the climbing way
With painful steps and slow...[5]

We want to assert that the promises of God are not extinguished by our darkest experiences. "The light shines in the darkness, and the darkness has not overcome it" (John 1:5) – or, "has not put it out"

---

4 John Henry Newman, The Dream of Gerontius

5 Edmund H. Sears, "It came upon a midnight clear".

– because it cannot. It did its damnedest to stamp out the light, but it could not. "For the Son of God, Jesus Christ ... was not Yes and No, but in him it is always Yes. For all the promises of God find their Yes in him." (2 Corinthians 1:19, 20)

We want to sing the resurrection psalm:

Even though I walk through the valley of the shadow of death,
I will fear no evil, for you are with me...

PSALM 23:40

As one modern song puts it, "for my God is with me. If my God is with me, whom then shall I fear?"* Or, indeed what shall I fear?

[* Matt and Beth Redman, "You never let go" © 2005 Thankyou Music (Adm. by worshiptogether.com songs excl. UK & Europe, adm. by kingswaysongs.co m tym@kingsway.co.uk www.kingsway.co.uk) with permission.]

We hope you will come on the journey with us.

Michael Wenham

CHAPTER 2

I wish...

Jozanne's Story

I wish I could take a long walk on the beach at sunset and feel the sand between my toes and the waves against my legs.

I wish I could jump from rock to rock with Luke and Nicole, catching rock fish with nets in the tidal pools on a beautiful sunny day.

I wish I could hike up the Outeniqua Mountain with Dave and the kids, and stop halfway up for a scenic picnic.

I wish I could bake cookies with Nicole, and giggle with joy as we decorate them with chocolate sprinkles and glazed cherries.

I wish I could tap my feet to the rhythm of Luke's guitar as he practises so diligently and enthusiastically for the Young Musicians' auditions.

I wish I could shoot goals with Nicole outside in the net. She loves to play netball, especially when she can be the goal shooter.

I wish I could stand and give Luke a big hug ... I'm sure he is almost as tall as me, or at least up to my chin.

I wish I could run my fingers through Nicole's beautiful blonde hair and help her tie her ponytails in the morning before school.

I wish I could straighten Luke's tie and collar every morning, and help him flatten that piece of hair he always seems to miss at the back of his head.

I wish I could get up in the middle of the night when the kids are sick and feverish, and when all they need is a cool facecloth and a comforting touch. I know Dave is there for them ... but I wish I could be.

I wish I could wake Dave in the morning with a hot cup of coffee and a soft kiss on the cheek. He brings me my tea every morning.

I wish I could cook him his favourite dinner, set the table beautifully and eat by candlelight like two lovebirds, while the kids visit ouma (grandma).

I wish I could play Nicole's karaoke game "Sing Star" with her. She has a beautiful voice and loves to perform. I am sure I could give her a go.

I wish I could be a cricket and hockey mom. I would love to sit by the sports field for hours, just to give Luke a big smile and a cheer when he looks my way "unintentionally" after he scores a goal or bats a big shot.

I wish I could paint Nicole's nails and give her a facial, do real girly things together like shopping at the mall, and having milkshakes, just the two of us.

I wish I could bake pancakes on a rainy day, or flapjacks and waffles for breakfast, just for the fun of it. The kids would say I am "the best mom in the whole wide world".

I wish I could help Luke when he puts gel in his hair before he goes to a friend's party, and "It's not because there are girls coming to this party, Mom."

I wish I could play "chopsticks" on the piano with Nicole, but I am sure she would play faster than me.

I wish I could dance with Luke, and show him how to hold a girl gently as you sweep her across the floor ... "Agh Mom, we don't dance like that!" he would say.

I wish I could wipe away Nicole's tears when her little heart is broken by an insensitive friend after a whole day of playing together.

I wish, I wish...

Jozanne Moss, May 2009

CHAPTER 3

Jozanne's diary

You never really understand a person until you consider things from his point of view – until you climb into his skin and walk around in it.

HARPER LEE[6]

Jozanne's Story

I was diagnosed with Motor Neurone Disease on Wednesday, 16 November 2005.

Saturday, 19 November 2005

I have decided to start writing down the things I feel in the hope that it will help me cope, but also so that one day, when this is all over, Dave, Luke, and Nicole can read it to remember me by, and also really to understand what I went through. Today, I feel great and at peace – but on Thursday my whole life seemed to tumble in.

I will start at the beginning – at least the beginning for me. In about June 2005, I started noticing

---

6 To Kill a Mockingbird, © Harper Lee 1960; Penguin Books, Harmondsworth, 1963.

that I couldn't run anymore. Now, I am not a runner by nature (built for comfort, not for speed – as my dad would say). We were having a school concert and, believe it or not, on all four nights of the performance, I forgot the same silly sashes the children wore and had to run back to the classroom to fetch them, literally moments before my kids went on the stage. It was during this running that I started to notice that my left leg didn't do what it was supposed to. It felt like it wanted to drag and I had to work extra hard just to get my one leg before the other. But with me being such a couch potato, I was convinced that it was because I was so out of shape and unfit. I was sure that a few sessions in the gym would change things. In any case, it wasn't affecting anything else. I didn't really tell anybody.

I don't know how much later, but I started to notice that, even when I walked, my left leg felt like it wanted to drag. I had to focus to pick it up, but yet again I was convinced that, if I had been more of a gym girl, this would not be happening. Remember, I am closer to forty than to thirty. I felt too embarrassed to really tell anybody, especially Dave, my husband. He was already on my case for not doing anything active. Well, time passed and I could feel that things were getting worse, slowly but surely. It was when I started noticing that my left hand seemed weaker (it couldn't do little things that I used to be able to do) that I told my mom. I have always been a mommy's girl! I was still convinced that a little bit of regular exercise would do the trick. It was my mom who eventually pleaded with me to go and see a doctor. Even then, I really wasn't urgent about it.

One day, both the kids were sick and I took them to the doctor. He examined them both and joked about whether there was anyone else in the Moss family that needed attention. I just happened to think that maybe I could mention to him what was going on. He examined me, watched me walk, and that is how it all started. He made me realize that maybe this was not nothing, especially when he suggested that I go to a neurologist. He could only get an appointment with the neurologist a month later. This made me feel more at ease. If this was serious the doctor would have squeezed me in sooner.

It took a whole month before I could see Dr Freda, the neurologist. On 20 September 2005 she examined me and immediately booked me for a brain scan (MRI) the very next day. I was thrown. What could it be? A brain tumour? The next day's MRI, thankfully, showed a perfectly healthy brain. It must be something else. Within a week I went for a spinal scan and a batch of blood tests. These too only showed how healthy I was.

By this time, I realized that the doctor was looking for signs of Multiple Sclerosis. I started to read up on the condition and it sounded terrible. The doctor seemed confused because the MRI was supposed to show lesions on the brain if indeed the diagnosis was MS. Next the doctor booked me for a spinal puncture to test the spinal fluid for early signs of MS. I was convinced it was MS. All the signs pointed to it, and I was starting to prepare myself mentally for this new turn that my life was going to take. When the results finally returned negative, I was still convinced I had MS and I had information from the Internet to prove that the spinal fluid test was a sensitive test and needed to be performed meticulously to get an accurate result. I didn't trust the outcome of the test.

Dr Freda decided that the next step was to do a MRI of my neck. I knew she wouldn't find anything, but I guess she had to cover all the bases. "A beautiful neck" were her words. At this stage I started feeling the anxiety that comes from uncertainty. Any diagnosis would do, I just needed something to be confirmed. I was also getting used to the idea of having MS. It seemed bad but I could live with that. In any case, someone in my family had it and they were still alive and kicking. Although their life had now changed, it was still a life of some sorts. Eventually, Dr Freda decided to send me to Cape Town for further tests. An appointment was made for me with a professor from the University of Cape Town.

On Wednesday, 16 November 2005, Dave and I left for Cape Town at about 10a.m. I was quite excited, hoping that at last someone would be able to tell me what was going on. I just wanted to know, so that I could educate myself, make the necessary adjustments to my life and carry on. (It all seemed so simple!) I was also looking forward to the five-hour drive, time I could spend with Dave in the car, real focused time. Time to talk about everything. Just the two of us. We hadn't had time for us lately, and hadn't discussed what was really going on. It looked to me as though Dave was in denial about everything. He still felt that, if I would just get some exercise, eat healthy foods, and get more rest, all this would go away.

The trip to Cape Town was nice and quiet. We couldn't really talk about IT. We just made idle chatter, but even that was fine. It felt like we were on holiday. We made good time on the road and arrived in Cape Town early. We decided to go to the Prof early and make sure we got all the paperwork done. After some searching we finally found the University of Cape Town Private Hospital at 3.55p.m. It all seemed very unassuming, like a real academic hospital. We were sent down the passage to room no. 2 and on the way there passed an odd-looking little man, probably a hospital orderly or something. I was feeling excited and anxious at the same time (a very weird feeling), but we arrived at room 2 and sat down to wait.

The odd little man we had passed in the passage came back and introduced himself as the Professor. Surprise! He definitely did not look the part, but I am sure he had lots of brains and experience. He asked all the usual questions, did the same examination as Dr Freda without the same professionalism, and after approximately 35 minutes let us sit down at his desk again. At this stage it did not look like he really had anything new to tell us. "Well," he said, "I have good news and bad news. The good news is that you don't have MS." I was overjoyed by the news, something solid. Dave and I looked at each other. We were so pleased; and I could see that look in Dave's eyes that said, "See, I told you so".

"Great, Professor! What is the bad news then?"

"Well, it could be blocks in the muscles. These cause the impulses from the brain to get blocked in the muscle and not to pass through, thus leading to weakness and spasticity. But my favoured diagnosis would be Motor Neurone Disease. I think it could be MND. There is just one more test we need to do called an EMG. This would confirm whether it is MND or not." We didn't know what he was talking about. He asked us whether we wanted him to be totally honest with us, even if it was bad news. "Of course!" we said.

The Professor explained that the neurones in my brain and spinal cord, that carry the messages from the brain to the muscles, were dying, and that slowly but surely I would lose the use of my muscles (and so limbs, etc). He assured me that my brain would not be affected, and when I expressed relief, he commented that maybe it is not such a good thing. This comment I did not quite understand at the time, but it now makes perfect sense to me. I asked the professor whether my breathing would be affected. He commented, "Not really so much," in a very uncommitted way. The Professor said we could listen to him dictating the report he was sending to Dr Freda, and that maybe we would have more questions afterwards. The report sounded mostly like Greek to us, except where he spoke about how he "favours" the diagnosis of MND. That word "favour" amused me at the time. It just seemed an unusual word to use under the circumstances, but I guess that was just his way of speaking.

Dave and I walked back to the car in a bit of a shock. What do you say? I guess we had some sort of diagnosis now, but what did it all really mean? Could the EMG test maybe prove that it was not MND? I broke down in tears, not because I really knew what was going on, but because so much emotion had built up to this one moment. I wanted certainty, and what I had now was still a measure of uncertainty. Dave held me for a while, and within moments I pulled myself together, and we headed for the traffic of Cape Town. We decided to go to the Strand and to get out of the rush of the city. We were able to get the last room at the Pavilion Hotel, overhanging the sea. It was all so beautiful. God was there; and from that moment on I could feel God's arms (his everlasting arms) around me.

Dave went to the shops and came home with sparkling wine and some snacks. In the meantime, I telephoned people close to me to tell them the news. When Dave got back we sat on the patio and watched the sunset as we drank a toast to something – I don't really remember what, but I know we wanted to celebrate something. It was wonderful and beautiful and moving. It was here that I realized I would not be alone and that I did not have to be scared. The evening was perfect. The next day we headed home.

I was eager to have that test (EMG – electromyogram) done as soon as possible because waiting was not something that I could do anymore. I telephoned my doctor to try to set it up for Friday, but was disappointed to hear that I could only have it done the next Thursday. So we were back to waiting!

I was eager to get home to see the kids, but also to jump onto the Internet for more information on this unknown disease that I might have. We arrived in George and went straight to my mom's house. It was when we stopped there and my parents came out the door that I realized something was terribly wrong. They looked in shock, as though someone had died. They had read the information on the Internet. We went in, and I asked my mom for the information they had read. I went into the study by myself and read. The shock was indescribable. This was not a disease: it was a death sentence. Everywhere, I read the life expectancy was between two and five years. That could not be: the kids are too young. How could I die now? Who would love them as much as I do or take care of them as well as I could? What would become of them? What now?!

I wasn't afraid for myself, or even Dave; we were OK. I am not afraid to die – how could I be? I knew and understood God's love for me and the grace that he has poured out in my life. Life with God is so much better than life here on earth. But my children! How do children so small grow up happily without a mother? This can't possibly be God's plan for them. How could it be? I know God wasn't looking away when I got this disease, but he has allowed it to happen; and I know that God does everything for the good of those who love him. Therefore, I do believe that there is a good reason why I have MND. I know that God does not give us anything that we cannot handle; so God must know that I can handle this. I just need to know and believe that. I believe that many people's lives can and will be impacted by this disease. My prayer is that I will be a beacon of light that shines God's love.

June 2007

Physically the disease is really starting to make things difficult for me now. My legs don't work anymore. I am able to stand, but not able to move my legs while I am standing. My right arm and hand are still in fairly good working order, but not my left arm and hand. This makes it still possible for me to shower myself. I sit on the commode, pull myself up by holding on to the bars that we had installed in the shower, and then I can still wash myself. When I am finished I can still dry myself and then flop back into the wheelchair that has been put in the right position with the brakes on! As long as I am holding on to something I am still able to do some things without help, but it's getting more difficult every day!

I know we have got Idie, my caregiver, to help me, but it's a big, vulnerable step to take, and I want to put it off until I really can't do it on my own anymore. To be so dependent on someone else, to be completely vulnerable in front of someone else! It's just so personal, and I just don't feel ready yet. "I can still do it! I will still do it on my own. I have to, and it's just too big a step to take!" I know the time will come when I have to hand over. It's probably here already, but I'm just not ready yet. The amazing thing about Idie is that, whenever I go for a shower, she's always nearby. Always conveniently busy with something right outside the bathroom door. I hear her moving around in my bedroom! No one sees my struggle and frustration behind the closed bathroom door. It's just taking me longer and longer to get through the routine of showering. I have realized that I am not washing as well as I should, and also not drying myself properly.

Then one morning I was in the shower again. My energy levels felt very low. I felt as if I was using every single bit of energy in my body to hold on to the rail with one hand and wash myself with the other hand. I was absolutely exhausted when I had to get out of the shower. I stepped out of the shower very carefully, holding on to the towel rail. I managed to get the towel off the rail, but my legs were shaking. I had to dry myself; I couldn't just flop into the chair. I tried as usual to get the towel around my shoulders with one arm, while holding on to the towel rail with the other. I tried numerous times. Then at one stage the towel dropped to the floor, and I just did not have the energy to pick it up and try to put it around me again.

I felt frustrated and exhausted at the same time. I could feel the tears were welling up in my eyes, a lump pushing up into my throat. I stood there, for what felt like hours, but it was probably just a few minutes. I knew the time had come. I had to call Idie to help me. With a very shaky voice I called. Her name had barely left my lips and she was there. Very discreetly and carefully, she half opened the door and stood behind it, so that she couldn't see me. I asked if she could help me. I pretended that this was not a big deal. I asked her very casually if she would just help me to dry myself quickly. With a big smile on her face and in the most natural way, she just took the towel and helped me. She helped me into my chair and then helped me to get dressed. It felt as if we had done this for many years already. I was so comfortable with her.

What a relief for me, what a breakthrough, what a huge step that I finally took! Even though I felt like I was losing a bit more of my independence, at the same time it felt like a mountain had been lifted off my shoulders. I realized that I had now reached a new stage in my illness.

The day continued and I was exhausted. So by late afternoon I was lying on my bed feeling vulnerable and emotional. A person doesn't realize how something like this can affect you emotionally. At about 4p.m. Idie popped her head around the corner to see if there was anything she could still do for me before she went home. She said her usual cheerful goodbye, and I almost felt uneasy. Surely there was something I could say. Did she realize what a momentous day it had been for me? I looked at her, and didn't quite know where to begin; but to my surprise, before I could say anything, she said, "Thank you so much for letting me help you today."

I was just blown away. I couldn't understand or believe that she was thanking *me.* Everything inside me was ready to thank *her.* It was a very special moment, and I thank God for loving me so much that he sent me someone like Idie. I am so grateful for her gentle nature, her care, her beautiful heart. What a profound moment! I am the one that was vulnerable and helpless and needed the help, but the one that served me so graciously is the one thanking me. I am continually blown away by God's love and the mystery that he holds and reveals to me in this time. And I am so incredibly grateful for his perseverance with me.

November 2007

Dave and I have just returned home from a week away. We went to Pinelake Marina, just outside Sedgefield, on the "Garden Route". The kids joined us from Friday night, and on Sunday my parents fetched them again for school on Monday. Pinelake Marina is a wonderful holiday resort that offers many fun activities, especially for the kids. We have been here a few times before, even when I was healthy, and we have built some fond memories together as a family. The weekend with the kids was no different. They spent hours in the pool, went boating on the lake, cycling around the resort, and jumped to their hearts' delight on the trampolines. We spent a great weekend together and the weather was beautiful.

On Sunday evening, after the kids left, it was just the two of us. We had the rest of the week to ourselves, but this was not going to be just another romantic holiday together. We had other plans and we came prepared. From the beginning of the illness I have wanted to make DVDs for the children. I wanted to leave special messages for them on special birthdays. I also wanted to tell them what I was like as a child, what they were like as babies, and how much I loved and enjoyed them. Kids want and need to know these things; I know I did. I loved hearing from my parents about their childhood, but also what I was like as a small child. I know I probably won't be around to see Luke and Nicole grow up, but I want to make sure that, as a mother, I will still be a part of their lives.

In the beginning, I thought that I would make a DVD every now and again, but it never materialized. I just never felt ready and always put it off for "one day". Lately, I have noticed that my speech is starting to change, ever so slightly, but I can feel it – as if my tongue is lazy and gets stuck when I say certain words. I have to work a little harder when I speak. People who don't know me wouldn't know the difference, but I know it's starting. We have decided to make the DVDs now, before it's too late. I want to sound like the real me when I leave my special messages for them.

So on Monday morning Dave and I woke up, ready to tackle this difficult task. While Dave set up the recording equipment, I made brief notes of more or less what I wanted to cover in my messages. When Dave was ready it was time to begin. He started filming ... I didn't feel comfortable at all. In fact, I felt so self-conscious, I was giggling like a little girl. I had too much nervous energy. I was trying too hard to sound natural, and instead came across fake. This is not what I wanted. Dave suggested that I just chat as though I was chatting to them. This was a lot harder than I ever imagined it would be and I felt so frustrated. Dave's phone rang and that broke the tension, but the phone call was to inform us that an old friend of mine's husband had committed suicide. They have two boys younger than

Luke and Nicole. I was devastated. No more filming that day.

Tuesday was very different. This time it was real. My friend's loss and pain became mine. When Dave started filming, I started crying. The thought of Luke and Nicole growing up without me became so real, and I now had the opportunity to leave them with something, unlike Linda's boys who will never really understand why their father left. What a privilege and special opportunity I have! Thank you, Lord. We made quite a number of DVDs in the days that followed and, although it was one of the hardest things I have ever done, it was also very fulfilling. It felt like a journey that I took with each one of the kids. My prayer is that it will be as special for them to watch the DVDs as it was for me to make them.

Another memorable thing about this past week is that, after the beautiful weather we experienced with the kids on the weekend, it started raining on Monday and didn't stop. It rained and rained, causing most of the holidaymakers to leave. The resort was left empty. By Friday, the flooding started and the lake rose up to completely flood the first row of chalets and the restaurant. Fortunately, we were staying in the second row. Some of the boats and hobicats were washed up onto the lawn and children's play area. The water level rose up to the horizontal bar that the swings are attached to. It was an unbelievable sight. When we finally left, there were no staff members in the resort, as most of them were unable to travel to work because of the flood. Reception was empty, and we just left our chalet key on the counter.

10 December 2007

This morning I received a big surprise and a special gift. At about 7.40a.m., a few of my friends arrived for a visit. I was still in bed, and knew something was up when they all sat around me on the bed looking very naughty. I asked them why they were here so early and reminded them that it wasn't my birthday for another nine months. They just all giggled. A few minutes later the phone rang and to my surprise the person on the other end of the line introduced himself as Nick Marais, the presenter of the breakfast show from a well-known radio station, KFM. I was live on air and caught completely off-guard.

Every year around December, KFM runs an initiative called *Christmas Wish* where they try to grant the wishes of people in special circumstances. My good friend Jeanette had nominated me for a Christmas Wish and my wish had been chosen to be granted. I couldn't believe it. We were given a luxury boat cruise for the four of us on board the MSC *Melody.* The cruise departs from Durban and travels up the coast to the Barra Lodge on the coast of Mozambique. This trip takes four days with all expenses paid. Included in this amazing gift are plane tickets for all of us, flying us up to Durban for the wonderful cruise. Wow, this is fantastic!

What a surprise! A few months ago, Jeanette asked me if there was still something I wished I could do. I have always wanted to go on a luxury cruise, but it was one of those dreams that I never thought would really materialize, especially not now. This is such a special gift, and to be able to experience it with the kids makes it even more precious. It is so important for me to build special memories with them. I know this cruise will be unforgettable. Thank you, Jeanette. Thank you, God.

January 2008

It's the beginning of the new school year, and the kids and I are very excited. I have always loved the beginning of a year. The newness of it, a new start, a new teacher, new books, new stationery! I love this time of year.

Beth and Errol (our pastor and his wife) have been a great support to us in our weekly meetings. We are able to discuss our circumstances with them and appreciate their outside perspective and support in the whole situation. It was at one of our weekly meetings that Beth told us about a situation at school. She had overheard one of the teachers telling another teacher how much she wanted us, the Moss family, to come and visit them on their farm "before Luke's mommy dies". I appreciated the thought but was shocked that a teacher would talk about me dying, so openly. I know she didn't realize that she could be overheard; I know that in her heart she wanted to support us, but just the fear of knowing that this could be overheard, and maybe somehow one child could tell another child and eventually tell my kids, "Hey, Luke, Nicole, I hear your mommy is dying."... I can just imagine the shock that my kids would feel having to hear this from someone else.

I guess in my heart I believe they know that this is coming, but I have no idea how children of nine and seven think. I don't know how they will deal with it, if they hear from someone else. Errol very supportively brings up the fact that it is time for us to tell them, and for us to explain to our kids that this illness that I have is terminal. Dave and I look at each other.

This has been the hardest part for me; and I have been putting it off. In my heart, I knew that we needed to have this conversation. Until now, we have been very open with them, by discussing the deterioration and the progress of the illness. But I have never reached a point where I have actually said that this is terminal, and explained to them that terminal means you die because there is no cure. It's very hard for me, but I know that they are right, and Dave and I look at each other with desperation. The tears well up in my heart and in my eyes. How do you broach this? How do you even bring up a topic like this? How will I be able to answer their questions? How will I be able to answer them in the way that they need to be answered? I pray in my heart, "God, please help me; please help us. Please give us the wisdom to answer these children, to comfort their hearts, to explain on their level what is happening to their mommy."

Dave and I never really get to a point where we make a decision on this. We know in our hearts it has to be done. But I don't know how. Do we do it together? Do we call a meeting? Do we bring it up as something serious? I don't know how, and I spend lots of time praying about it.

School will be starting in a week's time. We have all the new stationery and books, and Idie has been a great help in covering the books for me. Luke has been sitting at the table excitedly choosing pictures to put on his books. He's in grade 4 now. They are allowed to decorate their books, and put their own identity on them. With Nicole it is not the same, but she's very eager to mark all her stationery and to write her name on everything that belongs to her.

The kids and I are sitting at the dining room table; it's a fun time, the excitement and the exhilaration and nervousness of beginning a new year. The kids talk about who they think their teachers will be, and who they would like to have as their teachers. I share a little bit about when I used to start a new year. I say something funny – obviously by now my speech has deteriorated a little – and Luke bursts out laughing, teasing me. Something I pronounced in a funny way. We all laugh. It's been easy that way. I enjoy it when we can laugh together, even when it is about my illness, and it just breaks the tension! But suddenly, I realize this is a great opportunity to start talking about this topic.

"Have you noticed mommy's speech has been getting very bad?"

"Yes, mommy. Listen how you said that word."

We all chuckle. "Have you seen how this illness is getting worse every month? Do you remember that about a year ago I was walking with a crutch, and look, now mommy is in a wheelchair?"

"Yes, mommy. It's not very nice."

"Do you know that I'm not going to get better?"

"Yes, we know, mommy."

"Do you know that as this illness carries on it's going to go into my lungs, and it will affect my swallowing? It's going to affect all the muscles."

"Yes, mommy."

"I want to tell you something: this illness is going to cause my death."

There is silence in the dining room. Both kids are still carrying on with what they are doing, but they are quiet. I can feel my own tears welling up ... Please, Lord, I don't want to cry now. I want to get this out. I want to speak to them. Please help me not to cry. I don't want them to see my tears. I want them to hear my words.

"Mommy, when are you going to die?" Luke says.

"I don't know – when are you going to die?"

"No, mommy. No one knows."

"That's right, my boy. No one knows when they are going to die, but I do know that I'm not going to live as long as other moms do."

"So are you going to be a granny one day?"

"No, my love. I'm not going to get as old as ouma is."

"So, mommy, are you going to die in two years?"

"No, my love. I don't know if I'm going to die in two years. I know that this illness gets worse, and eventually I'll die, but no one knows when."

Nicole's very quiet. I am not even sure if she's listening. She's busy with her stationery and writing her name, but I am not going to push the issue with her. Luke on the other hand is looking very worried and panic stricken.

"Mommy, are you going to be here when I'm twenty?"

My heart feels like it has stopped inside my chest. "No, my boy. I'm not going to be here when you are twenty."

"OK, mommy."

There is silence. I don't want to cry, please Lord. I can feel the tears welling up.

"But you know what, kids. When I die, I'm going to heaven, and heaven is a much nicer place than earth, and that's where we all want to be. And when I go to heaven, there will be no more pain and no more tears."

"Yes, mommy. And you won't have to be in a wheelchair anymore. You will be able to walk and run and play," Luke says.

"That's right, guys. So I'm looking forward to going to heaven one day. I'm looking forward to being with Jesus."

It's quiet again. Nicole looks up from where she was busy, "Mommy, when you die, can I have all your jewellery?" I can't help bursting out with laughter.

"Mommy, can I also have your jewellery box?"

"Yes, of course, my angel."

"Oh good! I like your jewellery, and your jewellery box has a nice lock on it."

The conversation just carries on, and we laugh. We just start talking about other things. Both kids seem satisfied with the answers, and in my heart I feel so grateful and relieved. Thank you, God! Thank you for carrying me through this. I can't wait to tell Dave that we have had this conversation. We carry on working with books and stationery and pictures as though we have just had the most normal conversation. Inside, part of me is crying out in pain, but I don't show the kids. I have got mixed feelings of exhilaration and fear and anxiety for these kids. But I know that God will take care of them, now, and when I am not here anymore!

February 2008

It's early Friday evening. It's been a long week and we are all lying on the bed relaxing. I am in the wheelchair and Dave and the kids are lying on the bed. The TV is on and we are watching the news. I look at Nicole. She seems very upset, and I can see she's starting to cry.

"What's wrong, my angel?"

"Mommy, I don't want you to be ashed."

"What do you mean, you don't want me to be ashed?"

She starts crying even more. "Mommy, I just don't want you to be ashed."

"I don't understand, my darling. What do you mean?"

"When you die one day, you know, when they burn you – I don't want you to be ashed."

Before the diagnosis of my illness, we once discussed cremation, when my parents informed us that they wanted to be cremated. In that discussion, I had also mentioned that I wanted to be cremated one day. The kids weren't really part of the conversation, but they must have followed it. At the time, no one was dying and so I didn't mind that the kids were around. Nicole was obviously reflecting on this. I think a bit. Maybe she's worried about the flames and the body; maybe she's scared I will get hurt or will feel it. I try somehow to explain to her that, when you die, your soul leaves your body and goes up to heaven, but that your body doesn't feel anything anymore. I explain to her that when you get cremated or you bury the body, it's just a body. The person inside, your soul, has gone to heaven. But she's not satisfied with this answer.

"Mommy, I don't want you to be ashed. I just don't want you to be ashed."

I can't figure out why she's still upset. We talk about it a bit more. "But what do you mean, my darling? What are you worried about?" By now Dave and Luke are both listening. Nicole is really upset. Inside my heart is breaking, because how can it be that my seven-year-old has to worry and be upset about things like this at her age? I ask her again, "What do you mean, my darling?"

"No, mommy. I want a place where I can go and be with you when I need to see you; I want something that I can go to."

I finally realize what she means. When you are cremated, your ashes get scattered, and that's your choice. In her mind, if I was to be cremated, she would lose me forever. All she wants is something tangible, I guess, like a gravestone that she could go to if she needed to be with me.

My heart just breaks: this little girl of mine is already thinking about one day when I am not here and she will need me. I try to explain to her that I don't like graveyards; they seem so depressing. I try to explain to her that we will figure out a way for her to be with me; but I see that right now in her mind that will not be good enough and we agree to talk about it later.

I just want her sadness to go away. We lie there for a while in silence, just with the news making a noise in the background. But in my heart, I know that we have to talk about this again. I want her to understand that I will always be with her in her heart, that she won't need a place to go to, but I guess, if that is what she needs, I would love to have a bench in the garden or a special corner where, one day, she could go and sit and feel like she's with me. She's so young. It's so sad that she has to deal with this now.

March 2008

Family time is very important to me, especially meal times. We always try to sit down together around the table as a family, whether we are having pizza or Sunday roast with veggies. There, around the table, is where we have had the most amazing conversations. It's great to make time to hear the kids, to listen to what's important to them, and to find out what's happened in their day.

One particular evening, like so many others before, Nicole asked a question that took us all by surprise. She usually chats a lot and asks lots of questions, but this one was very unexpected. "Daddy, when mommy dies, are you going to get married again?"

Dave and I looked at each other. We didn't know what to say. There was an uncomfortable silence that felt like it lasted for ever, even though it only lasted a few seconds. In that moment, I felt quite nervous, and just wanted to put my little girl's mind at ease. "You know what, angel, even if daddy does get married again, I don't mind at all. I don't want daddy to be lonely. If daddy chooses to get married again, I would not be angry."

Dave looked at me. We had actually discussed this before; so at least for me this was not unknown territory. But to hear it coming from Nicole, knowing that this had been in her little mind, really caught us off-guard. Dave said, "My angel, I'm not thinking about or planning to get married again. That is in God's hands. Maybe I will; maybe I won't. But I want you to know, that I won't marry anyone that you and Luke don't like. I will first let you get to know her, and if you don't like her, I won't get married to her."

Nicole carries on eating. She doesn't seem at all fazed by what's just been discussed. It's only me and Dave that are feeling uneasy. A bit later Nicole looked up at us and said, with a mouth full of food, "Well, daddy, if you do get married, it better be to someone that I know veeeeery well." We all burst out laughing! The atmosphere is settled.

Aren't kids amazing? I realize that, right now, the kids need to know the practicalities. They need to know what the future holds, who's going to look after them, who's going to fetch them from school, who's going to be at home when they get there. Where are they going to live? Are they still going to have their own bedrooms? Who's this woman going to be that might come in my place? For us, these things might not seem important, but for them they are.

I see now that if I can comfort them at that level, it can really make a difference. I realize I can't protect them. This is a process Dave, myself and the kids *have* to go through. There is no way I can make them sidestep the pain that lies ahead. But I know there are some things I can do to make it easier. I am so grateful for the way the kids think, the simple way their minds work, the way they verbalize things, so uncomplicated. It makes it a bit easier for me.

19 May 2008

With a lot of effort, I can manage to get some food onto a spoon, if it's in a bowl. On a flat plate I end up chasing the food all around the plate. So with a bowl and a spoon, and some effort I can feed myself. But lifting the spoon to my mouth takes time and coordination. Often, just before I reach my mouth my arm starts shaking, and if it's not something that sticks to the spoon, I very quickly lose whatever I struggled to get onto my spoon. It's actually quite funny. I tell the kids, "Don't eat the way I eat. Your mommy is not an example." After every meal, we have to debrief the kids about how not to have table manners!

I know soon I'm going to have to be fed, but I love eating. So while I can still do it, and I still enjoy it, I will try my best for as long as I can. It's too difficult to put the spoon right into my mouth, and so I end up eating like a dog off the spoon. It's very funny, and I try to keep the humour in every situation. That's really not difficult to do. I think if anybody was able to see me they would have a bit of a chuckle. The kids certainly do, and I like to laugh with them. So eating has become quite an experience for me, and I must admit that my eating out days have come to an end. I don't want to embarrass whoever is with me: not everybody will see the humour in it. Dave and I celebrated our thirteenth wedding anniversary recently, and I would have loved to have gone out for dinner to a fancy restaurant; but we settled happily for a movie and double-thick milkshakes from McDonald's afterwards.

22 May 2008

It's Dave's birthday today. It's a Thursday, and normally I have a Bible study with Jeanette on a Thursday. Dave said I should go, and then he will pick me up at about 10.30, and we will go out for his birthday. We don't get a lot of time to do things together on our own anymore. We cannot just jump in the car and go do things anymore. A lot of effort goes into it, with the result we don't do much. So needless to say, I am very excited about my date with my husband! I am not sure what we are going to do. It is Dave's day, so it's his choice. He arrived at Jeanette's to fetch me in my favourite blue shirt. I looked at him and I felt very proud that he is my husband. I also had a blue shirt on, and so we looked like we were colour coordinated. We weren't quite finished with our discussion yet; so Jeanette asked him to join us. To my amazement, he sat there quite comfortably, the only thorn among the roses. And the contribution he made really impacted the whole group. I really felt so proud of him. At about 11 we got into the car, and Dave said he felt like watching a movie. I thought, that's great, that's something we always liked doing together.

We went to the mall, and looked at the movies that were showing. There wasn't a great choice, but it was Dave's day, so he could decide. He decided on *Indiana Jones,* a real adventure movie! We get some popcorn to munch on. Popcorn has always been a big treat for me; I could easily eat a jumbo popcorn by myself. I remember the days before the kids were born, when Dave and I would go to the movies on a Tuesday and each get a jumbo popcorn and devour it in no time! This felt like the old days. This time he gets me a kiddie's popcorn and a large for himself.

We are seated now, me and my popcorn and water. Dave's munching away at his popcorn. I soon realize I am really battling to get the popcorn to my mouth. Not just taking it with my fingers; my whole right hand has become very weak. Once I get the grip on the popcorn, my whole body has to lift my arm to my mouth. I know that I have been having difficulty feeding myself lately, but it never entered my mind that this would affect my popcorn eating.

Although the movie is action-packed, I struggle to keep my focus on it. I am having such a struggle with my popcorn that it consumes me. I am actually tired. I can feel my heart racing and I am out of breath, like someone running a marathon. The harder I try, the more exhausted I become. How can something that I used to enjoy so much become such a struggle, such an effort? I immediately decide to stop. I ask Dave to put the popcorn on the floor. Everybody around me is completely oblivious to my struggle. Inside me I feel that I have lost something. I can feel in my heart the mourning is starting. The mourning of a loss, the loss of the ability to do something that I used to enjoy so much, especially with Dave.

Eventually, I manage to get my thoughts off this and start to enjoy the movie, as much as I could possibly enjoy *Indiana Jones!* Not quite the movie club choice, but for Dave I will do anything! When the movie was finished, Dave asked if I want to take the rest of the popcorn home with me. Part of me wanted to hold on to this thing that I know I have got to let go of. I felt that I wanted to prove that I can still get it into my body, but deep inside I knew it was time to accept it and choose to let it go. That's why I threw it away! I tried to not show Dave how I felt, because I did not want to spoil his special day, but inside I was incredibly sad!

We decided to go for coffee. This was also one of our favourite things to do, because our first dates used to be coffee dates. I know the "Mug and Bean" well, because I often go there with Tara and my friends. So I feel quite comfortable there; they know how to make me comfortable around the table with my wheelchair. Dave offers to buy me lunch. I am absolutely thrilled because I love eating out. But these days eating with a knife and fork is a major effort for me. At home everybody helps me with my eating, but I have decided not to let Dave go through this in public. So I decline. But Dave persists; so I decide to have something I can eat by hand, like a toasted sandwich. I know my mood is different, and I can see that it is affecting Dave. He then says he does not feel like anything to eat, and so I decide I won't have anything either.

There's a bit of a strain on our communication, but I order Milo and Dave a coffee. As we are sitting there opposite each other, I think we both realize that things are very different now. Our usual going out, eating and having fun, has become a strain. Inside my sadness and frustration grew! I started feeling frustrated with Dave. I knew it was not his fault, but he just frustrated me. I did not know what he was feeling, and his lack of conversation with me made me feel like he wasn't interested in spending time with me. Immediately, my mind started running away with me. He was so busy on his phone and greeting others that he knew, it seemed that his focus was on everyone but me. I tried to make conversation, but I realized that every attempt was tainted by my feeling of sadness and loss.

At one stage, I tried to tell him how I was feeling, but as I started the tears were welling up in my eyes, and when he saw this he said to me, "Oh, please don't start crying now." That was a big blow to me. Here I was with the one person that I could just be myself with, and he was not interested in what I was going through. I felt bitter, sad, frustrated, and angry. After this, we had nothing to say to each other anymore. I so badly wanted this to be a special birthday for Dave, because with the way the illness was progressing, I couldn't see how we could do something like this on his next birthday.

I felt incredibly sad – so many losses, the loss of popcorn, the loss of eating out, the loss of spending a birthday with my husband. I felt a lot of anger and bitterness inside. I also felt rejected. I realize *now* that because of my change in emotion, Dave immediately thought he had done something wrong. He thought that if he did not make much conversation with me, he could just avoid getting into whatever it was that was hurting me. So for him his silence was to help the situation, but for me it was rejection.

June 2008

The value of us as humans is very often determined by the role we have in life. As a daughter you have parents and you're learning a lot. I just think of being a teenager, rebelling against authority, and I know that as a teenager you are very confused about your value as a person. As you grow older and you start to earn your own money, maybe you become a wife and mother, very often your value is determined by whatever role you are in. As a wife or husband, you are valued by your spouse, and that value is easily seen in the response you get from that person, the love that's returned when it's given out.

Then if you look at being a mother, that love is so easily returned by kids, and your value seems to increase so much more, because of the dependence that kids have on you. Mothers can do anything. Just the stroke of her hand or just a little cuddle can take away all a child's fears and stresses and worries. A mother is a perfect person, who can achieve almost everything in the eyes of a child. I remember, becoming a mother was one of the most amazing things for me. Being able to comfort, to nurture, to guide, to love, and to meet a child's physical needs, it's so incredibly rewarding, simply because of the child's response. I remember Nicole coming into our room in the mornings, and she would fling her arms into the air with a loud "ta da" and a big smile on her face.

I remember that feeling when the kids would want something and dad would go to help, but all they want is mom! It makes you feel wanted. Although you don't want to take anything away from dad, there is this feeling of satisfaction. What a fantastic feeling, what a privilege!

Another role that has given me value is the role of teacher. Knowing that in your hands, for a whole year, you have a group of children that you have such a huge influence on. In this year you can teach them, inform them, and mould them in a positive way. So being a teacher has added great value to my life as well.

But now as this illness progresses and I have less influence on others, I have started to wonder where will I find my value now? I cannot have influence on the school kids now, because I can't teach anymore. I tell myself at least I'm still a mother. But I cannot fulfil my role as a mother as I did before, because of the fact that physically I cannot do things for them anymore. I cannot come running when they call, or when they have hurt themselves. I have to rely on others to do that on my behalf. I look at my friends who are also mothers. How busy they are with everyday things! Fetching and carrying kids to school and back, to sport and back; fixing things, dropping off things, looking after the household, making food, etc. I cannot do any of this anymore; so it has become a real struggle for me to identify with my role as mother.

I had put my value in the role as a mother who could run a household, do projects with my kids, cook and clean, be a taxi to my kids. Now I cannot fulfil that role anymore, and I must admit this confused me in the beginning. I thought, "Well, what now? Where do I fit in, what is my purpose, what will my role be now? What do my children think of me, this mother that cannot do the things that they need for them anymore?" God's wisdom is so amazing. He teaches us in his word that we must have faith like little children. God wants us to simplify things, especially our thoughts. That is what I appreciate about kids; they tell it like it is.

Even though I can't put my arms around them when they fall or hurt themselves, I am still their mother. I am still the one they run to when they need to be comforted. I can still help with the homework, just being there and listening to Nicole's reading or Luke doing his oral. It's actually a very special time, lying on the bed together going through the homework.

Sometimes, it's hard for me to lie in bed in the mornings when I can hear Dave and the kids busy in the kitchen with the breakfast. I hear them laughing and doing the things I should be doing. This is when I have to remind myself that my value is not in the role that I used to play in their lives as a mother. My value comes purely from God, I am valuable because he created me and he loves me. I am incredibly grateful for this knowledge. I am so grateful that things can be simplified to that. It's a great comfort to know that even as my body deteriorates due to the illness, even when I won't be able to communicate with my children anymore, I know in my heart that I have a place in their lives as a mother, not because of the things I do for them, but because of the comfort they find in knowing that I am there for them. My prayer is that I will still feel like this in a year's time. But I know God is faithful, and I know he will meet those needs of mine and of my children.

November 2008

I am trying to write what I feel. I wish the computer could read my mind. It takes so long to type. I can only move my hand slightly, but it is enough to be able to use the mouse and the on-screen keyboard. This is a very tedious process, considering that I was once able to type quite fast. Thoughts come and go, but by the time I start typing so many thoughts have passed that I don't know where to start.

I am also starting to really struggle with my speech. The muscles of my mouth, tongue and soft palate are weaker, and this greatly influences the formation of sounds that form words. Sounds that are made in the front of the mouth with my tongue, like S, T, and R, tend to lose their sharpness or are absent altogether from words. So a word like "slipper" becomes "lipper". I just asked Dave: "What other words do I say funny?" and he just laughed. It came out as: "Wa udar wos do I hay funny?" I guess that was my answer.

I can still communicate my needs effectively, but having a flowing conversation is becoming very difficult and tiring. Not only do I struggle with forming certain sounds, I also get breathless quickly. The muscles between my ribs and my diaphragm, which control the flow of air from my lungs through my vocal cords, have weakened considerably.

November 2008

It was a Monday evening and on the 7 o'clock news we had just heard that Miriam Makeba had collapsed after a concert in Italy and died of a heart attack. The death of "Mamma Africa" is big news here in South Africa, and we all listen carefully to the news bulletin. With a puzzled look on her face, Nicole looks at me and asks, "Did she just fall on the ground and die? Was there any blood?" I then explain to her that usually when someone dies of a heart attack or stroke, there is no blood to be seen. In fact, a dead person looks like they are sleeping.

"Like this?" Nicole says, and demonstrates by bending her head to her shoulder and closing her eyes.

"Yes," I say, looking at her sweet little face as she pretends to be asleep. "Can death really be this beautiful?" I think to myself.

Luke is lying on the bed going through all the actions and sound effects that a ten-year-old boy could conjure up while pretending to be dying, and I see this as another opportunity to speak about my death in a comfortable and natural situation. I want to prepare the kids as thoroughly as I can. "No, Luke," I say, "it's very peaceful. Pretend you're sleeping."

He does and lies still like a toy soldier. "When I die one day, it will also look to you like I'm only sleeping."

"I don't want to see you when you're dead one day," Luke protests; and I quickly reassure him that he wouldn't have to if he didn't want to. But unlike Nicole, Luke is not comfortable with speaking about my death.

November 2008

It was a Wednesday afternoon and Dave was playing golf. When he played golf, he would only get home after 6p.m., and Idie would have to put an adult nappy on for me when she left at 4p.m. This was still a new step in the progression of my illness and it had been one of the more emotional steps to take. I remember the first time I had to put one on. I felt an intense sense of embarrassment and sadness, but all I could express was laughter. I giggled like a silly little girl at the mere sight of the adult nappy. It was so big. I don't know what I had expected, but this was not it. The way it made me feel was very unexpected. I wanted to cry out, but all I could do was laugh uncontrollably.

The times following this were, however, very different. I would mostly feel angry, with a deep sense of sadness, and would often cry during the procedure of putting on the nappy, after which I would once again, with God, surrender to my situation. Idie was always a very encouraging support to me. When I would cry, she would often try to make the whole situation a lot lighter by making a joke or something because she has a great sense of humour. But Idie always treated me with the utmost respect and dignity. I never felt embarrassed with her.

On this particular day, Idie had made one of my favourite dishes, spaghetti and mince, and although I so looked forward to it while she was cooking, I struggled very much to eat it. The mince, being granular, was all over the inside of my mouth, and difficult to gather into a ball with my weakened tongue in order to be swallowed. The spaghetti, on the other hand, was long and slippery, and kept on sliding to the back of my throat where it stimulated the choking reflex. As much as I wanted to, I just couldn't enjoy the meal. I was choking and spluttering all over the place. Idie suggested I use the food processor and, although the thought of processed spaghetti didn't really appeal to me, I agreed and she proceeded with it. The end product, I must admit, did not look appetizing but tasted exactly the same and was much easier to eat. And there we were – another step down the road of this tough journey I am on.

It was on this particular Wednesday afternoon that God showed me, again, how much he loves me and how he has provided me with everything I need to overcome and be victorious in my illness. When Idie had to put the nappy on for me, she commented on the fact that she had noticed that this time it didn't seem to bother me. I noticed it too. "So today I'm like a real baby," I joked. "I'm in nappies and I've started eating baby food." It was a silly thing to say, but part of me was still trying to cover up my embarrassment.

Idie smiled and with such love in her eyes she said, "No, together, you and I are still going to reach high places." She understood, and again God used Idie to love and encourage me.

10 January 2009

It is a warm Friday evening and we are having a braai (barbecue) outside. Dave loves braaiing and would probably braai everyday if he could. The kids love it too. It's always a great family time for us; even the dogs get to be part of everything. Nicole uses this opportunity to perform her many songs and dances to a captive audience; and the garden becomes her stage. Luke likes to show off his latest soccer or hockey manoeuvres. Then the sports field and stage soon clash. This is usually where Luke's attention turns to the fire. He likes to light the fire and then experiment with different objects to see how they burn. He has a very inquisitive mind. I love that about him.

This evening was no different. I was sitting in my wheelchair with my fancy new cup-holder stand, sipping on some cool drink, with our dog Amber leaning against my lifeless foot, hoping desperately to get a rub. Dave had just settled into his chair feeling confident that the fire he had made would not die. Nicole had just slumped to the ground from exhaustion after having performed the big finale from the *High School Musical 3* movie, with all its dance moves and more, and Luke was playing with the fire. He had burnt some leaves and twigs on the paving and was left with a pile of ashes, which he then proceeded to hammer down with a log.

"This is what mommy is going to look like one day," he said out of the blue, "one day when you are ashed."

"Cremated," I corrected him.

"Yes, mommy and I will be cremated, and daddy and Nicole will be buried," he said.

Immediately Nicole protested, "No, I don't want mommy to be cremated."

So, another opportunity was created for us to discuss this difficult topic in a natural and incidental manner. The kids continued to argue for a moment, and then Dave suggested that each child be given a chance to explain why they felt the way they did. Outspoken Nicole spoke first. It was clear that she still felt the same, and that she needed a place where she could go to mourn. I also realized from what she said that she had terrible images of a body being thrown into a fire and having to watch it burn. Dave explained again how the whole process worked, and Nicole seemed to understand better this time round.

Next, it was Luke's turn. Up until now, Luke had not expressed any opinion regarding cremation or any other topic about my illness. In the past, whenever Nicole would talk about death and my illness, Luke would just withdraw from the conversation and, although he didn't take part, I always hoped that he was listening. I didn't want to force him into any conversation that he wasn't ready for; so you can imagine my surprise when he spoke.

"I want you to be cremated because, if you were buried in the ground, mom, I would always feel that a part of you was still around. Then I would have to be sad every day. If you are cremated and we scatter your ashes," he said while scattering his pile of ashes into the air with a blow, "you will be free, and we can 'move on'. You have to 'move on', you know." He said this with such maturity, I was left speechless for a few moments.

"Yes ... yes, you're right," I said trying to sound composed.

Wednesday, 27 May 2009

My wonderful husband, Dave, has suggested I keep a journal. I started to write down what I was experiencing shortly after my diagnosis, but didn't keep up with it. Now, three years later, I think I might be ready to try again.

A lot has happened and changed in my life in the last three years, but I can't even imagine writing it all down. So I will just start with how I am doing now. I am in a wheelchair and I can't use my arms or hands. I have a feeding tube inserted into my stomach, but I am still able to eat food that has been puréed. My speech is very nasal and muffled, really only understood by those close to me and with great effort. I have a very special lady in my life who takes care of my every need. Her name is Idith Matolla, but I call her Idie. She is trained in home care nursing, but I know she is really an undercover angel sent by God.

Idie does everything for me, from showering, dressing and feeding me, to encouraging me, wiping my tears and laughing with me, and we do laugh a lot. I don't know what I would do without her, but God knew that, and that's why he sent her to me. Idie helps me on weekdays from 8a.m. to 4p.m., and every second Saturday from 9a.m. to 1p.m. So as you can see, I spend many unforgettable hours with her. If you add up all these hours a week it comes to about 42 hours, which leaves approximately 63 waking hours where I am left in the loving care of my amazing husband. Keeping in mind that Dave has a job, is both father and mother to Luke and Nicole, and has a household to stay on top of, you can see why he really is amazing.

As I am writing this, Nicole has accidentally shut her fingers in her bedroom door and she is crying. She comes running to me and I so wish I could just put my arms around her to comfort her. Instead, my limp and heavy arms just lie there on the armrests of the recliner I am sitting in. Nicole falls on her knees next to my chair and flops her head onto my chest. Her body shakes as she sobs – and I feel so helpless. It is in this painful moment that God chooses to encourage me. Through her hair and tears, Nicole lifts her head and looks at me, and all I can do is smile at her. Her face lights up as she says, "Mommy, I love your smile. You have a beautiful smile!" That was enough for her. She is so sweet and God is so faithful. He promises to never leave us or forsake us, and will never give us more than we can handle.

> *No temptation [hardship/struggle] has seized you except what is common to man. And God is faithful; he will not let you be tempted beyond what you can bear. But when you are tempted, he will also provide a way out so that you can stand up under it.*
>
> 1 CORINTHIANS 10:13 NIV

29 December 2009

Christmas has come and gone, and another year has whizzed by. It was a quiet Christmas with only the four of us and my mom. It felt empty without my dad at times, but at other times I forgot he even existed and felt guilty that I had forgotten about him. Chris and his family visited us for a few days before Christmas. We had a very special time with them. I found my brother again and we bonded. God created the opportunity for us to talk about the old days. I got the chance to say everything that was on my heart ... those things that you always hope to say one day and never find the right time to say. I love my brother dearly and got the chance to really tell him that. My heart is now one with his. What a privilege! I am so proud of him and what he has achieved in his life. I am proud of the man he has become with his warm and loving heart. I am proud of the father he is to Ashleigh and Amber, and the husband he is to Claire.

The kids loved having their cousins around. There is something very special about family; no matter how little you see each other, you always seem to be able to pick up from where you left off. Family are your people, "ons mense". Just doesn't sound the same in English. It really was a special time. It also gave Dave the chance to cement a friendship with Chris that will be so important for Luke and Nicole, when I am not here anymore.

I also received a visit from a very special friend, Lanel. We have been friends for almost sixteen years. When I first became ill, she was there with prayers, scripture, and words of encouragement. She visited from far a number of times and I often had the opportunity to share my fears and challenges with her, especially the fear of leaving my children behind to grow up without a mother. Last year, when we visited them, I still remember Lanel giving me the opportunity to share with her friends what God was teaching me through my illness about heaven and hope.

In March this year, Lanel's husband, Sarel, was tragically killed in a plane crash, and this friend who supported me so faithfully in my fears is now left to raise her two sons alone. Her visit with me now is such an honour. Even in her own pain, she is there for me and I am grateful. Her pain is still very raw and real, but when I look into her eyes, behind the pain, there is a hope that only comes from knowing Christ. Seeing how God is taking care of them, especially the kids, just strengthens my faith and hope for the future of my kids. I know that, when I die, Luke and Nicole will be fine.

On Christmas day, after the excitement of the day, Dave and I were lying on the bed watching the third Santa movie for that evening. The kids were watching in the lounge. We were all tired and just watching some mindless entertainment on TV. We have had a wonderful Christmas with delicious food prepared by my mother and, although it was a quiet Christmas this year, I know that the kids had a lot of fun. At one point in the movie that we were all watching, there is a hospital scene where a woman dies and her adult daughter is the one to break this news to the father. The father, who wasn't able to be at the mother's side because of work obligations, is very sad to hear about his wife's death. He is heartbroken and angry.

Then the scene changes again, as the movie continues. A few minutes later, Luke walked into our room crying. "What's wrong, my boy?" Dave asked.

"I don't want this to happen to mommy – then we will be sad for a very long time. I don't want to be sad for a long time," Luke replied.

This just broke my heart. I cannot prevent this pain. "When mom dies, you will be sad, but not all the time," I said. "You will still play with your friends, go to school and do all kinds of fun things. You will be sad at times, but not all the time. You don't have to be sad all the time. I wouldn't want you to be sad all the time."

He gave me a big hug, and I wished I could put my arms around him and hold him tight. I wish I could show him that everything will be all right, but I can't.

This Christmas has been difficult for me. To me it felt like my last Christmas. Even if I am still around in a year's time, I am sure I will be very weak and ill. I have based this assumption on the rate at which I have been deteriorating in the past four years. So feeling that this could be the last put pressure on me to make every moment special and memorable. But how can one possibly do that? How do you treasure every moment? Those around me were unaware, and being this sentimental just made me sad. I treasure every moment of every day with those I love. I think what I really wanted was for this Christmas to be memorable for Dave and the kids, but you can't do that. It will only be memorable one day in hindsight for them. I am actually glad that they didn't think the way I did, because that would have made this Christmas sad for everyone.

24 January 2010

I struggle with many things like not being able to move, play with, or even hug my kids. I cannot do my own hair, brush my own teeth, or even go to the toilet by myself. I cannot feed myself, or even chew my food. I rely on others for absolutely everything, which involves a lot of waiting and lots of patience. Generally, I think I do quite well at coping and overcoming these struggles. I don't think anybody has an idea of how tough things really are for me, but God is faithful and gives me the strength daily to carry on. I do have bad days, usually when I am tired, but thankfully not too often.

My latest struggle is the difficulty I have to speak. This is probably the hardest and most frustrating thing I have to endure. To add to everything, my breathing has become very strained; so to do even the slightest thing, like just being upright or keeping my head up, takes tremendous effort and energy. The act of speaking is probably the thing that takes the most of my energy, and therefore leads to me being a lot more tired.

A new thing I have also had to start coping with is muscle pain. I have lost so much of my muscle mass, leading not only to the loss of movement, which I expected, but also the strain of just keeping my limbs and neck supported on my body, which is something I didn't realize would happen. The obvious position of comfort and least amount of strain on any muscles, one would assume, would be flat on my back, but the problem then is that my throat muscles and tongue sink back, which then makes breathing harder but also makes it very difficult to swallow my saliva. This, in turn, makes me feel like I'm drowning, a very distressing feeling. The solution, therefore, is to lie with my head propped up quite high, but this leads to the muscle pain and spasms in my neck and shoulders. These spasms become so severe, especially on my left side, that my left cheek, right up to below my eye, goes hot and numb right up into my ear. I am really struggling with this at the moment and have moments where I just cry. This, I know, is very upsetting for the kids. I pray, and know that God is helping me daily to get through it. I don't like upsetting my children, but sometimes it is just too much for me to bear. I pray that God will protect their hearts.

Monday, 1 February 2010

We have had a good weekend, but even a good weekend is still emotionally painful. I have come to the conclusion that weekends are more painful than weekdays. I think the reason is because weekends are for family. In the week the kids have school, Dave goes to work and I spend my mornings writing and emailing. You don't have to be normal and healthy to do any of that. Afternoons are spent with the kids, where I have the privilege of listening to homework, Nicole's piano practice, Luke's guitar practice, or just catching up with the day's news. Nicole is the one who usually has all the news for me, and in the finest detail. Luke prefers to stick to one-word answers when asked about his day, but on rare occasions he comes home, filled with excitement and with a story to tell. I enjoy these times so much with my children. I don't feel like I am missing out on anything. However, weekends are different.

On weekends, the kids also want to do fun things like other kids, and I don't want them to miss out. So often they would go to the beach with Dave, or even for a hike up the mountain. They also like to go camping every once in a while, and are always sure to bring home lots of photos for me to see. I long to be able to go with them, but I will not stand in their way. I want them to have as normal a childhood as possible. They often get invited to other fun activities with friends. So I don't in any way feel that my children miss out on life.

This weekend, Nicole was invited to join a friend's family at their holiday home, on the beach, for the weekend. She was so excited to go. On Saturday, we gave them a call just to find out how things were going. They were having loads of fun, spending time on the beach and going for long walks. I was happy to hear that she was having such fun, but at the same time my heart was aching. She wasn't missing out – but I was. I want to be on the beach with her and I want to take long walks with her. I get very sad and the emotional pain I feel is almost a physical pain. It is the pain of loss, and it is very real. I am mourning the loss of motherhood. All my life I dreamt of being a mother, and now Nicole is at an age where she is starting to discuss things. I can see she is starting to question things and starting to form her own opinion about things. She is at a very beautiful age, though I suppose one can say that about every age. The point is, I want to be a part of it, and I can't.

But out of all of this also comes the good. Luke was at home all weekend, and God created a wonderful opportunity for us to have a very important conversation with him, and although I couldn't really say anything, I felt so much a part of it. Luke is a very special and sensitive boy. He has a very gentle heart, but as a result can be hurt very easily. This weekend, a friend of his had a birthday party and many of the boys in his class were invited, including Luke. On Friday night, however, only four of the boys were invited to sleep over at the birthday boy's house. Luke's four best friends were invited, but he wasn't. What a tough reality to face at any age! But when you are eleven, turning twelve soon, this reality can be very painful. At this age when being accepted is so important, it is even worse but, at the same time, a good time to learn about the harsh reality of life.

Luke came home from school on Friday, and within minutes I could see that something was wrong. He tried to look tough, but the minute I asked him if he was OK, he broke down in tears. "I feel so left out, mom." This boy who tries so hard to be big now became just a little boy again. I tried to comfort him, but his tears wouldn't stop. I couldn't hug him or hold him; all I could do was to tell him that it was not aimed at him personally. On a logical level that makes sense, but the reality is that nobody likes to feel left out. Luke bravely tried to pull himself together and hid his face in the cushion while he wiped the tears away. I am so proud of my brave, strong boy.

As the afternoon progressed, Luke became involved with playing with our neighbour's two sons. They are good friends and probably play more often than the school friends. They were having loads of fun, and so I suggested he invite them for his own sleepover. Their mother consented and the excitement grew. The sadness from earlier was something of the past. The boys spent the rest of the afternoon playing next door. At about 6.30p.m., round about the time that I was expecting the boys to come home for the sleepover, Luke walked in alone. I immediately noticed that something was wrong again. The tears came running down Luke's face, and with great sadness he told me that the boys weren't sleeping over anymore because they had been naughty all week and, because the two brothers were fighting, the mother decided to punish them, and not let them sleep over. The disappointment for Luke was just too much for one day.

Luke couldn't hide his feelings of rejection and sadness any longer. Tears were streaming down his face; mixed with the dust and dirt of the afternoon's playing. It made brown streaks run down from his eyes to below his chin. Again, I couldn't hold him or hug him, but this time Dave was home. We were sitting in the lounge and Dave took him in his arms as he shook with sadness. "Why doesn't anyone want to play with me?" he cried.

That evening turned out to be a very special and important time for the three of us. We talked about life not always being fair, and about things not always being what they seem. We spoke about truths and perceptions, how the world creates perceptions, but that the only truth is in God's word. We might think and feel accepted when we are chosen by our peers, but the truth is that our joy and confidence should come from God. What a difficult and abstract concept to learn and understand at any age, and something we will all learn continually! God provided us with the perfect opportunity to start teaching our son. God's timing is always perfect.

CHAPTER 4

Healing

It [faith] is a relational posture of trust that enables us to receive the will of God in a way that others can't. Faith is a pair of open hands.

PETE GREIG, ***GOD ON MUTE***

One subject that Jozanne is strangely silent about in her diary is healing. However, she would be an unusual twenty-first-century Christian if she had not thought about it and prayed for it. She would be unusual too, if she had not been urged to have "faith" for her healing. Well, she's not unusual! In my experience, most Christians with chronic or terminal illness encounter well-meaning encouragement to pray for their healing. After all, Jesus' ministry was full of miraculous healings, and he is "the same yesterday and today and for ever" (Hebrews 13:8). Nothing is impossible with God, we are told. So, sometimes the unspoken implication, or suspicion, is that our continuing illness must be the result of a lack of faith or sin. Pete Greig, one of the founders of the worldwide 24/7 Prayer movement, in his outstanding book *God on Mute,* vividly recalls the assault on his faith when his wife Samie suddenly has a life-threatening seizure as a result of a brain tumour. He stands outside the hospital door among all the cigarette stubs of the many like him who have waited impotently while the medical staff struggle to save their loved-ones' lives.

> *...out here, standing in the smokers' ash under a grey sky, I felt closer to God and talked to Him as best I could. I told Him I trusted Him, repeating the same childish little phrases over and over again like a monk muttering the rosary: "Please make her better ... Heal her, Lord ... don't let there be a problem...."*[7]

However, of course, healing is something with which Jozanne did have to engage with early on. In her first email to me (and other friends) she wrote about her own wrestlings with the issue.

Jozanne's Story

I was diagnosed with Motor Neurone Disease about three years ago. Motor Neurone Disease (MND), also known as Lou Gehrig's Disease or Amyotrophic Lateral Sclerosis, is a rare condition caused by the breakdown of the nerve cells in the brain that control the muscles. It is a disease that gets worse over time. It affects the cells that control voluntary muscle activity including speaking, walking, breathing, swallowing, and general movement of the body. Nerves dealing with feeling to the skin aren't affected; so there is no

---

7 Pete Greig, God on Mute, Survivor, Eastbourne, 2007, page 38.

numbness or pins and needles. The parts of the brain dealing with intelligence and awareness are not affected. Unfortunately, there is currently no medical cure, and life expectancy will depend on how symptoms progress.

In the years that I have had MND, the word "healing" has come up in many conversations and with many different reactions. When the professor in Cape Town made the diagnosis of my illness he used phrases like: "there is no cure for it", and "there is nothing we can do for you". A few days later, I was confronted with words like "terminal illness" and "incurable disease", as I read all the medical information I could find about MND on the Internet. My first response to all of this was shock and then numbness. I could not conceptualize what that meant, considering the fact that at the time the only symptom I had was a lazy left foot. There was no pain and no suffering; so how could I possibly be dying? But the doctors were sure, and a final test called an electromyograph confirmed the professor's diagnosis.

Almost immediately, my mind, trained through Scripture to be obedient, focused on the knowledge that God has the power to heal me completely. With news of my illness reaching family and friends, I received the same words of encouragement: "We are so sorry to hear, but remember, God is faithful and he can heal you. You just have to believe and not doubt." Many, many people I know and even a whole lot I don't know prayed for my healing and are still praying. I am very grateful and humbled by this outpouring of love.

For a while, I clung on to every bit of "faith" I had, and refused even to consider the fact that I might not be healed, even though the thought often flashed through my mind. I had, from the beginning, found complete peace in knowing that my life, and my illness, were in God's hands. But I guess the big question was, "*Would* he heal me?" I did not want to "doubt" and would deliberately push "negative" thoughts out of my mind. But I started feeling uncomfortable when people would say that God *"will"* heal me. Not because I didn't believe he could, but because I wondered *why* he should. Why me? Why should I be healed, and not the three-year-old boy who died of cancer?

All around me people were trying to help with advice on the latest remedies, cures and eating plans, and I put some to the test with great hope in a positive outcome. I tried my best and was prepared to do whatever was necessary for health and healing. "Am I taking the right amounts?", "Have I detoxed enough?" and "Am I doing enough?" were some of the anxieties I started to face. I started feeling guilty when I didn't stick to my new health plan, and I realized that my focus on healing made me miserable. I became more concerned about what *I* was doing and lost sight of what *God* could do. It was then that I decided to give it all up, just to let go and completely hand over to God. I am not saying that one should not follow a health regime; it just wasn't a good thing for me. If God is in control of my life, he would most certainly also be in control of my healing. It was a very freeing thought. Thinking and praying like that allowed me to be completely surrendered to whatever the outcome may be.

I studied the Bible and found that God speaks a lot about healing his people/nation in the Old Testament. God wanted them healed from their sinfulness and disobedience. This refers to spiritual healing.

In the New Testament, Jesus heals many people and performs many other miracles. These miracles are awesome in the eyes of the people and confirm Jesus as the Christ. Jesus also gives his apostles the authority to perform miracles as they go out to proclaim the good news.

> *When John heard in prison what Christ was doing, he sent his disciples to ask him, "Are you the one who was to come, or should we expect someone else?" Jesus replied, "Go back and report to John what you hear and see: the blind receive sight, the lame walk, those who have leprosy are cured, the deaf hear, the dead are raised, and the good news is preached to the poor. Many people believe and are saved."*

MATTHEW 11:2–5 NIV

It is so evident that Jesus was concerned about the physical well-being of people, by the way he fed and healed them, but ultimately his concern is for their spiritual well-being.

I started sharing my new-found peace and insight from God with others and was faced with varied reactions. While some people understood, others thought I had given up completely and lost all hope. With grave concern and out of love, some people approached me with words and scriptures of encouragement. "Don't lose hope now!", "What about faith? Jesus died so that you can be healed." This scripture was often used:

> *But he was pierced for our transgressions, he was crushed for our iniquities; the punishment that brought us peace was upon him, and by his wounds we are healed.*
>
> ISAIAH 53:5 NIV

I know that I have been healed spiritually because of Jesus' wounds.

I was given a number of books to read on faith and healing, but my conviction that nothing happens to me without God knowing about it or it being within his will is strong. I know that God allowed this illness to come my way, and I know that he has a purpose and a plan with it. "But God's plan is to prosper you, how can it be his will for you to be ill?" people have said.

"'For I know the plans I have for you,' declares the LORD, 'plans to prosper you and not to harm you, plans to give you hope and a future'" (Jeremiah 29:11 NIV). Yes, God's plan is to prosper me by giving me hope and a future, and he has already done that. Jesus is my hope and heaven is my future. That doesn't mean I don't believe that God would want to heal me; it just means to me that God has already fulfilled his promise. He doesn't have to heal me. I am the clay and he is the potter. Who am I to demand anything? "'O house of Israel, can I not do with you as this potter does?' declares the Lord. 'Like clay in the hand of the potter, so are you in my hand, O house of Israel'" (Jeremiah 18:6 NIV).

God can and does heal, but everything God does is for his glory. If my life brings glory to God in my illness, then so be it. On the other hand, if God wants to glorify himself by healing me, then that will also be his choice.

> *As he went along, he saw a man blind from birth. His disciples asked him, "Rabbi, who sinned, this man or his parents, that he was born blind?"*
>
> *"Neither this man nor his parents sinned," said Jesus,* "but this happened so that the work of God might be displayed in his life."
>
> JOHN 9:1–3 NIV

No amount of effort or will on my part will change a thing. All I can do is put my trust in the Lord, not only for me and my life, but also that of my family, because the Word says: "And we know that in *all* things God works for the good of those who love him, who have been called according to his purpose" (Romans 8:28 NIV).

God has put eternity in our hearts, and I have truly come to understand that we were not created for this world. As children of God, we are just passing through. This is not our final destination. Heaven is.

> *In this you greatly rejoice, though now for a little while you may have had to suffer grief in all kinds of trials. These have come so that your faith – of greater worth than gold, which perishes even though refined by fire – may be proved genuine and may result in praise, glory and honour when Jesus Christ is revealed.*
>
> 1 PETER 1:6–7 NIV

So how am I doing now?

I am definitely growing weaker in my body. My speech is also deteriorating rapidly. I have a full-time caregiver who feeds me and looks after my physical needs. I am faced daily with the frustration of not being able to do anything for myself, even little things like scratching an itch or adjusting uncomfortable clothing. I have to rely on others to do all this for me. But within this frustration and total dependence, God is teaching me how to be completely surrendered to him. He is drawing me closer to him in a way that I have never been before. Despite my situation, God has surrounded me with everything I need to be victorious in this life.

He has given me his peace:

Rejoice in the Lord always. I will say it again: Rejoice! Let your gentleness be evident to all. The Lord is near. Do not be anxious about anything, but in everything, by prayer and petition, with thanksgiving, present your requests to God. And the peace of God, which transcends all understanding, will guard your hearts and your minds in Christ Jesus.

PHILIPPIANS 4:4–7 NIV

He has given me hope:

Therefore, since we have been justified through faith, we have peace with God through our Lord Jesus Christ, through whom we have gained access by faith into this grace in which we now stand. And we rejoice in the hope of the glory of God. Not only so, but we also rejoice in our sufferings, because we know that suffering produces perseverance; perseverance, character; and character, hope. And hope does not disappoint us, because God has poured out his love into our hearts by the Holy Spirit, whom he has given us.

ROMANS 5:1–5 NIV

He has given me an amazing husband, who has had to take over everything in our household, and who supports me in a way I could have never imagined. I also have two beautiful children who are adjusting so well to our circumstances, and who will one day be amazing adults because of what God is teaching them now. God has also surrounded us with an incredible support structure. And we are so grateful for all the prayers, meals, encouragement, and support we receive continually.

So you see, I feel like the lucky one, because I feel completely loved by God.

CHAPTER 5

The Kingdom, healing and faith

Jesus was going around "doing the kingdom", healing the sick, cleansing lepers, feeding the hungry, he was celebrating at a party with all the wrong people, transforming people's lives and saying cryptic things such as: "Let me tell you what the kingdom of God is like."

TOM WRIGHT, BISHOP OF DURHAM

Jozanne's experience of having her faith questioned or being urged to have "more faith" is one with which many will identify, whether patients or those observing them. It is a fear above all, which believers with an incurable disease recognize, "Am I not healed because of my lack of faith?" For the connection between faith and healing is unmistakable in the New Testament.

What about Jesus?

Jesus launched his ministry with proclaiming the kingdom and healing many, in fact all who came to him. But then, throughout the gospels, we meet individuals whose healing involves faith, either on their own part or on the part of someone else.

The haemorrhaging woman has faith to touch the hem of Jesus' robe (Luke 8:48). The blind beggar outside Jericho keeps shouting, "Jesus, Son of David, have mercy on me!" and is rewarded with the affirmation, "Recover your sight; your faith has made you well" (Luke 18:38, 42).

Jesus responds to the faith of the four friends who let the paralysed man through the roof (Mark 2:5). A centurion comes to plead for his servant who lies paralysed at home. "Truly," says Jesus, "with no one in Israel have I found such faith" (Matthew 8:10), and the servant is healed. The woman from the Lebanon region desperately argues with Jesus for her daughter's healing. "Then Jesus answered her, 'O woman, great is your faith! Be it done for you, as you desire.' And her daughter was healed instantly" (Matthew 15:28). Conversely in Nazareth, "he did not do many mighty works, because of their unbelief" (Matthew 13:58).

On all sides, it seems, faith plays a part in healing. Jesus himself teaches that it is vital. A desperate father has brought his demonized son to him, who experiences life-threatening seizures, but Jesus is not there. He's with John, Peter, and James on the mountain of Transfiguration. And so the remaining disciples try to help. After all, they have had experience of this sort of thing before, on their mission trips. However, they fail; and when Jesus returns, the father turns to *him.* Mark records Jesus challenging his faith: "All things are possible for the one who believes," and the man's instant passionate reply: "I believe; help my unbelief" (Mark 9:23, 24).

> *And Jesus rebuked the demon, and it came out of him, and the boy was healed instantly. Then the disciples came to Jesus privately and said, "Why could we not cast it out?" He said to them, "Because of your little faith. For truly, I say to you, if you have faith like a grain of mustard seed, you will say to this mountain, 'Move from here to there,' and it will move, and nothing will be impossible for you."*
>
> MATTHEW 17:18–20

Here, Jesus introduces a third party for faith in addition to the sufferer, and the asker: the person imparting the healing must have faith.

This, I think, is the key to the many times when Jesus heals people where apparently no faith is being called upon: for example, with the demonized, or with Peter's mother-in-law, the widow of Nain's dead son, and the paralysed man by the Pool of Bethesda, who seems to have no hope, let alone faith (Luke 4:19; 7:13; John 5:6–9). John 9, as Jozanne noted, tells the story of the man blind from birth. Jesus heals him so "that the works of God might be displayed in him" (9:3). What are the "works of God" which are about to be demonstrated? First, John, as he narrates the event, shows Jesus as the *revelation* of God himself: "As long as I am in the world, I am the light of the world" (9:5). The increasingly sharp divergence between the Pharisees and the formerly blind man ends with him not only recognizing Jesus as a prophet but also worshipping him as God. Ironically, as the Pharisees have earlier encouraged him to "Give glory to God", so John shows him doing just that, and Jesus accepting his worship. This is the "Son of Man" of Daniel 7:13, 14, the human incarnation of the invisible God and representative of his people, to whom "a kingdom is given". Secondly, we learn more of the *nature* of God in the encounter, notably his authority, demonstrated over disease and disability, and in judgment, dividing the spiritually sighted and blind. And we see his compassion in healing the man in the first place, and then later in seeking him out when he has been ostracized from the synagogue community. Don't be misled into thinking that this is Jesus making a point or providing a case study. At its core, this is Jesus caring about an individual in need of what only he can give him, healing and an encounter with his Creator – in other words, compassion and grace.

It's not an isolated case. It reflects the nature of Jesus. It is what Matthew comments on in describing Jesus' Galilean ministry:

> *And Jesus went throughout all the cities and villages, teaching in their synagogues and proclaiming the gospel of the kingdom and healing every disease and every affliction. When he saw the crowds, he had compassion for them, be-*

cause they were harassed and helpless, like sheep without a shepherd. Then he said to his disciples, "The harvest is plentiful, but the labourers are few; therefore pray earnestly to the Lord of the harvest to send out labourers into his harvest."

MATTHEW 9:35–38

As often happens, they become the answer to their own prayer!

What about the early church?

In the early church's life we meet all these elements involved in healing, faith on the part of the sufferer, of others, and of the healer, as well as concern for the glory of God. Paul and Barnabas, on their journey through Turkey, are preaching at Lystra, and Paul sees a man "who was crippled from birth and had never walked. He listened to Paul speaking. And Paul, looking intently at him and seeing that he had faith to be made well, said in a loud voice, 'Stand upright on your feet.' And he sprang up and began walking" (Acts 14:8–10). We almost miss the detail of Paul's "loud voice", which presumably was to draw attention to the healing and the ensuing message he intended to proclaim about the kingdom. Only it misfired! The townsfolk hailed him as the Greek messenger god.

Peter had more success, after the healing of the lame man at the Beautiful Gate to the temple in Jerusalem.

> *Why do you wonder at this, or why do you stare at us, as though by our own power or piety we have made him walk? ... His name (Jesus, the Author of life, whom God raised from the dead) – by faith in his name – has made this man strong whom you see and know, and the faith that is through Jesus has given the man this perfect health in the presence of you all.*

ACTS 3:12, 16

Here is the harvest for which Jesus had told his disciples to pray for workers, which began on Pentecost, the Festival of Shavuot, or the wheat harvest.

The New Testament may or may not provide the pattern for contemporary church life, in particular in the area of healing. After all, times have changed. By the grace of God medical science has advanced. Maybe Jesus' *modus operandi* is a sign of his time. That does not seem to be his view, however.

During his ministry Jesus sends his twelve apostles and a larger group of disciples to carry out his mission of proclaiming the kingdom and healing the sick. His final commission is to "make disciples of all nations, baptizing them ... and teaching them to observe all that I have commanded you. And behold, I am with you always, to the end of the age" (Matthew 28:19,

20). The "long" ending of Mark 16, verses 9 to 20, provides an expansion of the commission, which includes the sign of healing.[8] The book of Acts paints a picture of continuity between Jesus' and the early disciples' ministry. They preach the good news of the kingdom and there were accompanying signs, which authenticated their message and demonstrated the presence of the king. Sometimes, healings seem to occur with a similar frequency to Jesus' own miracles. After the shocking deaths of Ananias and Sapphira, we read of many signs and wonders done by the apostles, even to the extent of people being brought to be healed by Peter's shadow! "The people also gathered from the towns around Jerusalem, bringing the sick and those afflicted with unclean spirits, and they were all healed" (Acts 5:16). Philip causes a sensation in Samaria, with "many" exorcisms and "many" healings (Acts 8:7). Individuals are physically restored to life, such as Dorcas (Acts 9:40) and Eutychus (Acts 20:9).

And obviously such things were not the preserve of the privileged few, or even the original disciples. Gifts of healing and the working of miracles are among the variety of Spiritgifts endowed to the Church "for the common good" (1 Corinthians 12:9, 10).

---

8 The long ending's authenticity as part of the original gospel is disputed, but it seems to me at least to be an early commentary of how the church understood the commission.

Is anyone among you suffering? Let him pray. Is anyone cheerful? Let him sing praise. Is anyone among you sick? Let him call for the elders of the church, and let them pray over him, anointing him with oil in the name of the Lord. And the prayer of faith will save the one who is sick, and the Lord will raise him up. And if he has committed sins, he will be forgiven. Therefore, confess your sins to one another and pray for one another, that you may be healed.

JAMES 5:13–16 ESV

James is not directing his letter to a particular church that we know, but giving general guidelines to churches. His teaching about healing within the church community does not envisage it as a passing phenomenon, nor indeed as being extraordinary, since he goes on to cite Elijah who "was a man *with a nature like ours"* (James 5:17).

It's common to imagine that miracles such as healing just "faded away" as time went on, or as the apostles died. However, this is not the case. We read of them continuing in church life. For example, in about A D 180, Irenaeus who was Bishop of Lyons, writes about Christians still exercising the same gifts, including driving out demons, healing the sick, and even raising the dead.[9] About 140 years later, at the

9 Adversus Haereses, Chapter 32.4

other end of the Mediterranean, Eusebius wrote about evangelists in his history of the church: "The Holy Spirit also, wrought many wonders as yet through them, so that as soon as the gospel was heard, men voluntarily in crowds and eagerly, embraced the true faith with their whole minds."[10] I suspect that, far from fading away, there have always been miracles accompanying the gospel of the kingdom, even if they have not always been recognized or believed. Of course, the good news has not always been proclaimed consistently.

What about today?

If miraculous healings are not just a thing of the past, why do we not see more of them? Is it because we lack the vital ingredient of what James calls "the prayer of faith"?

Well, saluting such figures as Smith Wigglesworth on the way, skip 1800 years or so, to the present day. In *My Donkeybody,* I cite examples I have met of miraculous, or at least unexplained, healings. Many working in Christian ministry, I suspect, could do the same. We pray for healing and occasionally, to our surprise and joy, something quite out of the ordinary happens. More often, quite routine (though far from ordinary) medical treatment leads to recovery, or to

---

10 Ecclesiastical History 3.37, translated C.F. Cruse; Baker House Books, Grand Rapids, 1994.

deterioration and death. However, it's not mostly in the developed world with all its sophisticated medical resources that we find New Testament patterns of church life and experience. I suspect that is because the developed "first" world is the twenty-first-century equivalent of Nazareth, where familiarity had bred contempt and scepticism. As well as modern medicine having thought God's thoughts after him, and discovered many remedies, we have also replaced faith with structures and systems.

> *On a recent Sunday morning as we all sang and danced in our sandy green tent, an older Makondi woman with a beautifully tattooed face gave her life to Jesus. She ran up in the dust and told me how her daughter who was completely out of her mind was healed in church the Sunday before. Another lady jumped and screamed, "I can see, I can see!" as Jesus opened her eyes. She too wanted to follow the Lord!*[11]

This is just one cameo from what this book calls "A Year of Miracles". Clearly, it is far from unusual in the life of the Iris Ministries, based in Mozambique. I cite the ministry of Heidi and Rolland Baker, merely, because it is the one which I have come across and which has impressed me for its authenticity. Heidi comments on Jesus' encounter with the lawyer who

---

11 Heidi and Rolland Baker, The Hungry Always Get Fed, 2007, New Wine Ministries, Chichester, page 68.

came to test him with the question, "What must I do to inherit eternal life?":

> *If we love God with all our beings, we will live! If we do this, we will see revival. If we do this, the Gospel will go forth. This is the simplicity of Jesus' message. The power of God, the presence of God, the multiplication of the Gospel, is as simple as this: a physical demonstration of the love of God. We have overcomplicated our message, thinking we were being wise. We have analyzed the Gospel to death until it doesn't work any more! We have made it so intensely difficult to understand that we have theologized, theorized, and strategized ourselves into a corner. We have not understood that the Gospel is as simple as this: love, love, love, love, love!*[12]

Teisa Miller, who also works with Iris Ministries, writes:

> *In Mozambique, the average person has no access to medicine or quality health care. If someone gets sick, the believers fervently fast and pray, knowing Jesus is the only source of hope and deliverance. And guess what? Many people get healed. Not all instantly, and some people do not get healed at all. But, when believers continually turn to Jesus with expectant, de-*

---

12 ibid, page 49

pendent hearts the kingdom of heaven comes to earth![13]

It seems that there is certainly a connection between healing and faith. But that's not all. There's also a link between healing and God being given glory. In fact the glory of God and the coming of his kingdom are the prime focus of attention. Those who have experienced the ministry of Heidi Baker, as I have on one memorable evening, will bear witness to the consuming sense of the love of God. Healed or not (as in my case), I was left in no doubt that God loved me – which in view of my innate mortality ultimately matters more than an extended life. In that moment, I glimpsed the glory, the nature, of God.

It's no coincidence that healings are more in evidence at the kingdom's cutting edge than in its comfortable hinterlands.* We feel we can do without. We can prove God's existence without his intervention (which is an odd view, as Christian faith depends on history-changing interventions of cosmic proportions). Effectively, we don't need him, either for ourselves or for himself. After all, some would argue, asking God to intervene and heal is the antithesis of trust. Yet, in fact, it seems to me to be a biblical paradox that praying for healing and accepting suffering are *both* attitudes of faith.

(* For more about the kingdom of God on earth, see Chapters 7 and 24.)

---

13 ibid, page 137

CHAPTER 6

Surrender

Pain insists upon being attended to. God whispers to us in our pleasures, speaks in our consciences, but shouts in our pains. It is his megaphone to rouse a deaf world.

C.S. LEWIS[14]

"Surrender" is a very unfashionable word, with its connotations of accepting defeat. And yet oddly there's an old revivalist hymn which has come back into popularity, with the opening line, "All to Jesus I surrender". "Surrender" originally means handing something back to its rightful owner or to the person who has a claim to it. In warfare, the archetypal image is the desperate waving of the white flag at the Alamo. The original meaning is the more helpful. The sense in which Jozanne used "surrender" in her next email is similar. It is more than an acceptance of suffering, though it is that; it's more like Job's extraordinary declaration of faith: "Though he slay me, I will hope in him" (Job 13:15). Or, as a young song-writer, Chris Steventon, has recently put it, "We surrender to you,

---

14 The Problem of Pain, HarperCollins, London, 2002.

Lord – is our battle-cry."[15] It is a learned unconditional trust in the goodness of God's purposes *for me,* which enables us to continue with our spiritual war till our final breath.

Jozanne's Story

When I was initially diagnosed with Motor Neurone Disease, I had two choices: I could either accept it or fight it. But what does it mean to "fight" it? And what is the "it" that I am supposed to be fighting? MND is a rare illness and medical science has not yet discovered the cause of it or a cure for it. So what do I fight and how do I fight it?

Now, many would argue that my battle is spiritual and that the forces of evil are attacking me. I would agree with that to a certain extent; illness and disease were not created by God in the Garden of Eden, and only entered the world through sin and the fall of man. So yes, it is evil and not good, but God had a plan from the beginning. He sent Jesus to the world to overcome death for us, and by his blood shed on the cross, we have access into eternal life with God. In other words, God's plan was to restore his original creation.

---

15 Into His likeness, Copyright © Chris Steventon, 2009, with permission.

Jesus came, and has returned to heaven, to be with the Father and to prepare a place for us. The battle is won! We are set free and, as followers of Christ, will have eternal life with God when Jesus returns. But for now, we still live in this broken world with our broken bodies. The world is ravaged by disease, illness and death, and we continually face hardships and struggles, but the battle has been won and Christ has been victorious. Daily, all over the world, people are turning to Christ and finding the hope that sustains us here on earth. Our lives here on earth are but a breath compared to the eternity we will spend with God one day, and so I have to ask myself, "What is it that I still want from God, if (through Jesus) he has already given me everything?" No, I should rather ask, "What is it that God wants from me?" The answer to this question has become very clear to me: God wants us to know him and to trust him.

Knowing God does not mean knowing about God. Many people know many things about God. To really know God is to have a relationship with him, like a child has with a parent. This kind of relationship is built on complete trust.

So now that I am faced with this terminal diagnosis, I have to hold on to what I have come to know about God's character, and then I have to trust him, even when things don't make sense. I know, when I got this illness, God wasn't looking away by accident and missed it, or lost control of my life for that instant. No, God was exactly where he always is ... on his throne, in complete control of his entire creation and all his children.

> *The Lord himself goes before you and will be with you; he will never leave you nor forsake you. Do not be afraid; do not be discouraged.*
>
> DEUTERONOMY 31:8 NIV

> *Therefore go and make disciples of all nations, baptizing them in the name of the Father and of the Son and of the Holy Spirit, and teaching them to obey everything I have commanded you. And surely I am with you always, to the very end of the age.*
>
> MATTHEW 28:19–20 NIV

Based on this knowledge, I have complete peace with, and faith in God's will for my life. I might not understand it, but I do trust it. I am completely *surrendered.*

And this is where I thought my lesson in surrender ended ... but was I wrong!

Surrendering to God in the face of adversity is one thing (like choosing the strongest army to fight the enemy), but it is a totally different battle when it comes to surrendering your own will to that of God. This, I am discovering, is a daily battle and is based not on feelings but on choice. Daily surrender to God is an active choice you make in light of your relationship with him and your trust in him. Another word for this, I think, is *obedience.*

In my life, God is using so many situations to teach me to surrender and trust. In some I have been victorious, but so many times I have failed. Many times it has been obvious that I just needed to surrender, but often I have been stubborn and slow to change, usually to my own detriment. All in all, I have been grateful for his love and patience, like a father, wanting his child to grow and mature, but all the while drawing me nearer and nearer to him.

With my illness, there are many times that I have had to surrender, like when I had to start using a crutch and then a wheelchair. I tried to carry on walking for as long as I could, which in itself is not a bad thing, but when it causes distress to the rest of the family it becomes a matter of pride. Dave feared the day that he would receive a phone call at work to say I have been injured. He warned me, but I always laughed it off until, one day, Dave got that call. I had fallen in the house and hit my head on the kitchen counter. My head was cut open and I had suffered concussion. Luckily, my neighbour found me and could call Dave. After some stitches and a week in bed I was fine again, but realized that with the distress I had caused Dave and the kids it wasn't worth holding on to *my* desire to walk. I trusted God and surrendered to a wheelchair.

As the illness progressed, I started losing the fine motor skills of my hands. This coincided with Nicole starting grade 1. There were many things I could no longer do, and I had to surrender to that. One thing stands out as being particularly difficult for me to let go. Being in school meant that now Nicole had to have her hair in ponytails. I tried and tried, but could just not get it right anymore. Like so many other things, Dave gladly offered to take over yet another of my tasks. Being a man (and a balding one, at that) Dave had no idea how to tie ponytails. I tried to explain and he tried his best, but they still came out all skew and crooked. This became an endless source of frustration for me because I wanted those ponytails to be done my way. This one silly thing started to cause so much stress in the mornings, that I couldn't even watch Dave when he tied Nicole's hair, without feeling anxious and frustrated.

I realized I had to surrender. I thought I *had* to trust Dave, and in doing so I would be trusting God. For me, that meant trusting that Dave would get it right. That was difficult because the facts were clear: Dave was not good at tying hair. But God has used this very silly situation to teach me a very important truth about surrender and submission. Surrender in this situation meant trusting God in the outcome. The fact was that Dave would never tie hair the way I did, but I could always trust the outcome, and the outcome was always the same: Nicole's hair was in ponytails and, therefore, she adhered to the school rules.

Submission or surrender in a marriage is the same. My husband might not always make the "right" decision, or do things in the same way as I would, but I can always trust God with the outcome, whether a good or a bad outcome. This I know, because I know God: and God never changes. He is faithful in all situations.

And we know that in all things God works for the good of those who love him, who have been called according to his purpose.

ROMANS 8:28 NIV

It's been two years since then, and Nicole has learned to tie her own hair into beautiful ponytails. My illness has, unfortunately, also progressed to a point where I am virtually paralysed and unable to do anything, but day by day I am learning to be more and more surrendered to my circumstances, and therefore to God. It isn't always easy, but it has brought me closer to the Father with an intimacy that brings me so much joy. This intimate relationship, I believe, has only been possible because my will or my "self" has had to die. Only once we take ourselves out of the picture are we able to have close fellowship with God.

This, then, is how you should pray: "Our Father in heaven, hallowed be your name, your kingdom come, your will be done on earth as it is in heaven..."

MATTHEW 6:9–10 NIV

CHAPTER 7

So where does sickness come from?

Badness is only spoiled goodness.

C.S. LEWIS[16]

A question which Jozanne raises is, if everything which God created is good, what is the source of sickness and disease? It is clearly not made by God, even if he allows it.

A good place to begin would be by asking what Jesus thought. There is a hint of his view when he encounters a woman bent double "who had had a disabling spirit" and heals her in the synagogue on the Sabbath. He describes her as "a daughter of Abraham whom Satan bound for eighteen years" (Luke 13:11, 16). Jesus' compassion for the woman is clear. Indeed, he invests her with the utmost dignity, "daughter of Abraham". There is no sense of her being punished by God for her sin. Nor does Jesus perform an exorcism; he merely says, "'Be freed of your disability.' And he laid his hands on her, and immediately

16 C.S. Lewis, Mere Christianity, HarperCollins, London, 1997.

she was made straight, and she glorified God" (verses 12–13).

Her condition seems to be more a symptom of the fake kingdom of Satan, whose citizens, far from being free, are "bound". It is this usurped power that Jesus refuses to recognize in the wilderness temptations. The disciples have partially glimpsed the point when they are hoping for the restoration of the kingdom "to Israel" after the resurrection; but they are yet to discover the reality, the magnificent universal kingdom of Jesus' reply: "It is not for you to know times or seasons that the Father has fixed by his own authority. But you will receive power when the Holy Spirit has come upon you, and you will be my witnesses in Jerusalem and in all Judea and Samaria, and to the end of the earth" (Acts 1:7, 8). This is not the political restoration of Israel from Roman domination; this is the universal restoration of God's kingdom in his creation – a project so vast the poor disciples might be forgiven for not grasping it!

I doubt whether we ourselves perceive its scope. It's turning round the whole of human history, from its primeval course, to an almost inconceivably beautiful rightness. The figure of Jesus stands at the tipping point. Indeed, incredibly, this first-century Palestinian Jewish enigma *is* himself the tipping point. No wonder John Milton calls on the Holy Spirit for help as he writes:

Of Man's first disobedience, and the fruit

Of that forbidden tree, whose mortal taste
Brought death into the world, and all our woe,
With loss of Eden, till one greater Man
Restore us, and regain the blissful seat...[17]

We have every reason to believe that Jesus would have recognized this view of the origin of sin, and "all our woe", ranging from pain, sickness and death to man's inhumanity to man and environmental disaster.

Lost paradise

Genesis 3 in effect tells the story of humankind's loss of the kingdom of God, or the kingdom of heaven. Human beings listen to the voice of independence over the invitation to trust. The voice of independence comes from "the serpent", the subtle tempter, disguised in nature, who later in the Bible is to emerge as Satan. Although his fate is pronounced: "He [the woman's offspring] shall bruise your head", this is not the end of the serpent's activity; "and you shall bruise his heel" (Genesis 3:15). Snapping at humankind's heels, doing anything to take human eyes off the source of life – that is Satan's realm. He distracts humankind, but he cannot destroy us. Adam and Eve, however, have lost Paradise, the Garden of Eden where they walked and talked with the Lord God in the cool of the evening. God has not stopped caring

---

17 John Milton, Paradise Lost 1.1–5.

for them; he makes them garments of skins. But they can no longer have a part in his kingdom, because of their fatal choice. As the prophet later puts it: "your iniquities have made a separation between you and your God, and your sins have hidden his face from you so that he does not hear" (Isaiah 59:2). They have surrendered themselves as hostages to their impulses and survival instincts. And thus sin is ever present, "crouching at the door" (as Cain is told). "Its desire is to have you, but you must rule over it" (Genesis 4:7). It has soon becomes apparent why God "commanded" the prohibition which the serpent suggested was such an infringement of rights. The alternative to obedient trust is untrammelled licence, and all our woes.

Or maybe, we think, there is a third viable option, and that is creating a society which legislates away that licence, which controls those selfish impulses and survival instincts by means of laws. The biblical example is, of course, the people of Israel, to whom the Law is given. There's no mistaking that the Law is given by God. The engraving of the ten commandments on the tablets of stone is "the writing of God" (Exodus 32:16); as it were, they receive his seal of approval. However, for all the experiences of his grace to them (such as the exodus from Egypt to the promised land) and for all the advantages of the Law and the prophets, even God's chosen people are singularly unsuccessful in this alternative way. No amount of legislation, it appears, is able to create an ideal society. Attempts to create a brave new world are doomed to failure. No amount of legislation will silence the serpent. He is already outside the Law.

Satan is an outlaw with pretensions. He has no loyalty to the king. He aspires to the throne. Paul describes him as "the god of this age" (2 Corinthians 4:4); and that is the limit of his sphere of influence. But within those limits he delights to bruise those creatures made in God's image: to make them live with eyes directed at creation level, not Creator level.

Regaining paradise

The Gospels show Jesus' ministry of mercy as a rescue mission from the kingdom of darkness, which was allowed into God's creation at the fall of humankind at the dawn of time. The Greek word σωζειν (sozein), usually translated as "save", can also mean "rescue", and even "make well" (Luke 17:19). When John the Baptist in prison sends two messengers to enquire whether Jesus is "the one who is to come", Jesus' reply is to demonstrate the wholesale rout of the forces of darkness.

> *In that hour he healed many people of diseases and plagues and evil spirits, and on many who were blind he bestowed sight. And he answered them, "Go and tell John what you have seen and heard: the blind receive their sight, the lame walk, lepers are cleansed, and the deaf hear, the dead are raised up, the poor have good*

news preached to them. And blessed is the one who is not offended by me."

LUKE 7:21–23

That last sentence may seem curious in context. Is Jesus really telling his cousin off for having doubts in prison? That seems so out of character that I think it's unlikely. I suspect it *is* the general comment that it sounds like – the observation that all these good events, these signs of God's kingdom coming on earth as in heaven, are not universally welcomed. They are met with a mixture of reactions: some welcome them for what they are, evidence of God's love for human beings and his new world; others treat them with scepticism, and even downright hostility. The kingdom of darkness, inspired by the "father of lies" (John 8:44), will not readily admit defeat.

The same, of course, applies to the decisive turning point of the tide. Some recognize the cross as God buying back his world through the act of ultimate sacrificial love; some dismiss it as untrue and irrelevant. This is what Jesus refers to as "my hour" (John 2:4) or "my time" (John 7:6, 8; Matthew 26:18). Most often he calls it "the hour". On the Tuesday before Good Friday, some Greek pilgrims come looking for him. He tells his disciples, "Now is the hour for the Son of Man to be glorified" (John 12:23), and he proceeds to talk about his rapidly approaching death: "Truly, truly, I say to you, unless a grain of wheat falls into the earth and dies, it remains alone; but if it dies, it bears much fruit" (John 12:23–24). "The hour" will look like defeat – the death of the one figure who consistently stood and routed the forces of evil. And yet it isn't. As two days later Jesus prays to the Father, he recognizes that it is to be the moment of victory:

> *he lifted up his eyes to heaven and said, "Father, the hour has come; glorify your Son that the Son may glorify you, since you have given him authority over all flesh, to give eternal life to all whom you have given him. And this is eternal life, that they know you the only true God, and Jesus Christ whom you have sent."*
>
> JOHN 17:1–3

The outcome of "the hour" will be two things: the possibility of eternal life and the restoration of knowing (not knowing about) "the only true God" in his mysterious completeness.

The significance of "the hour" is nowhere more graphically demonstrated than in the exchange on the crosses between Jesus and the repentant thief. "And he said, 'Jesus, remember me when you come into your kingdom.' And he said to him, 'Truly, I say to you, today you will be with me in Paradise'" (Luke 23:42–43). Paradise, the place of God's presence, where he walks and talks with us, is about to be restored. And a man with no qualifications is about to be admitted. For him, death is not the end. In his end is his beginning. The primeval curse, the curse of Eden, has been reversed.

The kingdom is coming. On the day of Pentecost, Peter announces its arrival in the four events of the death, resurrection, and ascension of Jesus, and his gift of the Holy Spirit:

> *this Jesus, delivered up according to the definite plan and foreknowledge of God, you crucified and killed by the hands of lawless men. God raised him up, loosing the pangs of death, because it was not possible for him to be held by it ... This Jesus God raised up, and of that we all are witnesses. Being therefore exalted at the right hand of God, and having received from the Father the promise of the Holy Spirit, he has poured out this that you yourselves are seeing and hearing.*
>
> ACTS 2:23–24, 32–33

And so, Peter announces the beginning of the new age. No longer is the message, "The kingdom is near"; it is "The kingdom is *here"*. "Let all the house of Israel therefore know for certain that God has made him both Lord and Christ, this Jesus whom you crucified" (Acts 2:36).

The ongoing battle

Thus the question that gnaws away at the Christian with a medically incurable condition is, "Where is that kingdom?" and, as Jozanne has discovered, it bothers many who surround us, who want to see it impacting on us.

I suspect it was in Oxford lectures by my brother, David, in 1986–7, that I first encountered the "Already-but-not-yet" understanding of the kingdom of heaven, originally clarified by the American scholar, George Eldon Ladd. I found it illuminating in reading the Gospels and the Acts. For, while it has been argued that the miracles were merely signs, i.e. proofs of the truth of Jesus' claims, they were more than that: they were demonstrations of his authority in the here and now, and precursors of what we will one day see in full reality. The most helpful illustration of this, which I believe came from the Lutheran theologian, Oscar Cullmann,[18] was the comparison with D-Day and VE Day in Europe in the Second World War. 6 June 1944, when the Allies invaded Normandy, could be considered the decisive turning point of the war, spelling the end of Hitler's domination of Europe. Unconditional surrender, however, did not happen until nearly a year later, after many costly battles and many thousands of casualties. Victory in Europe was eventually declared on 8 May 1945. Similarly, Christ's death on the cross and resurrection was the decisive turning point in human history. Final victory is assured; the enemy knows his fate is sealed. However,

18 Oscar Cullman, Christ and Time, SCM Press, London, 1962.

the war is not yet over. Battles remain to be fought. The kingdom has arrived – but is not yet here. When we pray, "Your kingdom come, your will be done, on earth as it is in heaven," it is more than a pious future wish; it is a vital present commitment. We live between D-Day and VE Day.

This seems to me to ring true with our experience as Christians. As one friend of mine used to say, "We have been saved; we are being saved; we shall be saved." In a different context, Paul says, "For now we see in a mirror dimly, but then face to face. Now I know in part; then I shall know fully, even as I have been fully known" (1 Corinthians 13:12). We see signs of the kingdom now, because the kingdom has broken into history with Jesus, but only when he returns will we see it in its completeness. Then the new heaven and the new earth will be here – but that's for later!

But how exactly is illness linked to sin, to the primal human instinct for independence and survival? Is sickness a punishment for or a consequence of sin? (We have already seen Jesus contradicting blame in two individual cases, and so we talking here about the general prevalence of disease.) In the primal account of the fall in Genesis 2 and 3, God warns that the consequence of eating from the tree of the knowledge of good and evil will be death (2:17). This duly happens when Adam and Eve are excluded from the Garden of Eden, and therefore from access to the tree of life. When God pronounces judgment on Eve, he predicts multiplication of pain in childbirth, and for

Adam, pain and sweat in mere survival. And so "death and all our woe" enter human existence. As the Biblical narrative unfolds, it becomes clear that neither sin nor its consequences are confined to Adam and Eve. It is a shared, in fact an inherited, experience. Universal death and universal sin are part of the same package, concludes St Paul: "...just as sin came into the world through one man, and death through sin, and so death spread to all men because all sinned" (Romans 5:12). Elsewhere, he terms this "bondage to corruption", with which the whole of creation has been infected and from which it longs for release (Romans 8:21).

That sin and disease should be linked is not surprising. We are aware of some links. For example, we know about illnesses which are stress-related or induced by environmental factors. Even something as common as overwork (perhaps Adam's "sweat of your face") can lead to physical collapse. In the case of the disease we know best, "to date, research suggests that most forms of MND are likely to involve a combination of a wide variety of genetic and environmental risk factorss" (MND Association website, 2009).

To put it crudely, we smoke to satisfy our narcotic addictions, and the result is disease and death. Our greed becomes need, and we end diseased and dying. Because we can, we burn fossil fuels to travel faster and faster, not regarding the pollution. We want power, and power corrupts, as far as nuclear war. And we have only just begun! On a global scale, disease and sin clearly are connected. However, Jesus' example cautions us against drawing such a connection in the case of individuals. Even when the correlation may seem obvious to us, for example, in someone whose liver is sclerotic through alcohol, we need to ask who else sinned. We might find it is also the society of which we ourselves are a part.

CHAPTER 8

When it doesn't make sense

In a dark time, the eye begins to see

THEODORE ROETHKE[19]

"So now that I am faced with this terminal diagnosis, I have to hold on to what I have come to know about God's character, and then I have to trust him, even when things don't make sense," says Jozanne. She is not alone in wrestling with things that don't make sense.

One of the most remarkable personal revelations of this century was the publication of Mother Teresa of Calcutta's letters to her spiritual guides. The nun whose remarkable compassion and apparently serene faith had won her the Nobel Prize for Peace was suddenly discovered to have spent her years of caring for the poorest of humanity with a constant sense of the absence of God. "I am told God lives in me, and yet the reality of the darkness and coldness and emptiness is so great that nothing touches my soul" (quoted on the CNN website, 7 September 2001). She continues: "Where I try to raise my thoughts to

19 Theodore Roethke, In a Dark Time.

heaven, there is such convicting emptiness that those very thoughts return like sharp knives and hurt my very soul. Love – the word – it brings nothing." Whether this long-lasting crisis of faith was triggered by the mass suffering she met in the slums of Calcutta can be only a matter of speculation, but it would not be surprising if it were.

And others have felt the absence of God. The founder of the Passionist Community, Paolo Francesco Danei (St Paul of the Cross, 1694–1775), experienced fifty years of desolation and darkness when he felt as though God was far from him. The great Baptist preacher of the nineteenth century, Charles Spurgeon, was prone to terrible depression. "I often fall deep into the valley of despair," as he put it. The poet, William Cowper, suffered severe bouts of manic depression and tried to commit suicide three times. The title of his hymn, "God moves in a mysterious way", is *Light Shining out of Darkness.* Martin Luther became so desperate that he would hide himself away for days. The story is told of his wife, Katherina, trying to break its grip by dressing in black. When he asked her who had died, she replied that no one had but she thought God himself must have died from her husband's mood. Katherina Luther quite aptly expresses the feeling of distance from God, which many believers are alarmed to find in themselves. They know that it is not true; they know it's probably a result of something in their own circumstances. However, old certainties fly out of the window and God *feels* absent.

Then faith comes in. All Job's feel-good factors are systematically and comprehensively removed: his prosperity, his family, and finally his health. The archetypal righteous man is left, scratching the sores all over his body with a broken piece of pottery, in the ashes. His wife can no more understand his disinterested faith than can Satan. Surely things don't make sense? She asks him, "Do you still hold fast your integrity? Curse God and die." But he said to her, "You speak as one of the foolish women would speak. Shall we receive good from God, and shall we not receive evil?" (Job 2:9–10). Job does not curse God; he does not deny his existence. But neither does he deny his own physical and emotional agony. He seems to shout at God:

I loathe my life; I would not live forever....
Leave me alone, for my days are a breath....
What is man, that you make so much of him...
and that you set your heart on him...
visit him every morning and test him every moment?

JOB 7:16–18

Job's arguments are an astonishing mixture of brutal bluntness and touching trust, summed up in the extraordinary statement: "Though he slay me, I will hope in him" (Job 13:15). He probably means that he's prepared to take the risk of a meeting with his Almighty adversary, as it feels. It's a measure of his desperation *and* of his faith that the Judge of all the earth will do right. Battered by the platitudes of his comforters, which are calculated only to increase his desolation, sitting among the ashes, scratching away at his open sores, he still doggedly declares: "I know that my Redeemer lives, and at the last he will stand upon the earth. And after my skin has been thus destroyed, yet in my flesh I shall see God, whom I shall see for myself, and my eyes shall behold, and not another" (19:25- 27).

His three friends, with their "comfort", only exacerbate his pain, as he knows that they are not being honest; they are actually biased in God's favour – as if God needs that! His frustration is God's elusiveness. "Behold, he passes by me, and I see him not; he moves on, but I do not perceive him" (9:11). He is in the dark night of the soul. He cannot get near God, or so it feels:

> *Behold, I go forward, but he is not there, and backward, but I do not perceive him; on the left hand when he is working, I do not behold him; he turns to the right hand, but I do not see him. But he knows the way that I take ... God has made my heart faint; the Almighty has terrified me; yet I am not silenced because of the darkness, nor because thick darkness covers my face.*

JOB 23:8–10, 16–17

He is experiencing an overwhelming sense of the absence of God. "Oh, that I knew where I might find him..." (23:3) must be one of the most poignant heart-cries of a person of faith.

Job's dark night does come to an end, when God shows up, not in conventional religious tameness, but out of a whirlwind. One would love to know what God's tone is in his two panoramic revelations of creation at the end of the book. Is he angry? Is he battering this man who has dared to complain? Is he reasoning or making a case like a barrister? Has he a twinkle in his eye? Is there tenderness in his voice? All he does is to pose a whole series of questions, which reveal both the infinite variety of the created universe and the very limited scope of human understanding. "And the LORD said to Job: 'Shall a faultfinder contend with the Almighty? He who argues with God let him answer it' "(40:1,2). After the first unanswerable barrage, Job sensibly declines to argue – and then receives a couple of parting shots zooming in on Behemoth and Leviathan (probably the hippopotamus and the crocodile), familiar enough creatures of nature and yet thoroughly impenetrable mysteries to the contemporary mind. Job's final declaration is worth quoting in its entirety, because it is the ultimate statement of faith of someone for whom things have desperately and painfully "not made sense":

Then Job answered the Lord and said:

"I know that you can do all things,
and that no purpose of yours can be thwarted.
'Who is this that hides counsel without knowledge?'
Therefore I have uttered what I did not understand,
things too wonderful for me, which I did not know.
'Hear, and I will speak;
I will question you, and you make it known to me.'
I had heard of you by the hearing of the ear,
but now my eye sees you;
therefore I despise myself,
and repent in dust and ashes."

JOB 42:1–6

Far from being a grovelling admission of defeat, this is a conscious, almost joyful, realignment of perspective. This is the God whom I know, who is great, all-powerful and way beyond my comprehension, and confronted by him I am dust and ashes. I am out of my depth. All I can do is worship. In the words of the children's song, "Our God is a great big God" (Nigel and Jo Hemming), or rather more profoundly, "In a dark time, the eye begins to see" (Theodore Roethke, *In a Dark Time).*

For Christians, of course, the creation, glorious though it is, is not the ultimate revelation of who God is – or what he is like. The truly remarkable fact about

Jesus, who is that revelation, is that he experiences intense physical and spiritual pain and separation from God, all consequences of our primal sin. And this has a particular significance for those experiencing the dark valley with its temptations to doubt and despair, to doubt that God is in control, and that he is, indeed, love, and to lose hope not only for this life but also for life to come. At its deepest, at its darkest point, it descends to the blackness of God's absence. For us, this is perceived. For him, the cry, "My God, my God, why have you forsaken me?" is how it really is (because for him perception is not different from reality: see Mark 15:34). "For we do not have a high priest who is unable to sympathize with our weaknesses, but one who in every respect has been tempted as we are, yet without sin" (Hebrews 4:15). What the psalmist saw by faith, we know is true, because Jesus has pioneered the way: "where shall I flee from your presence? If I ascend to heaven, you are there! If I make my bed in Sheol, you are there!" (Psalm 139:7,8)

CHAPTER 9

Communication

It's good to talk.

BRITISH TELECOM ADVERT

Jozanne's Story

I started struggling with my speech in about August 2008. It was very gradual, and started with just a slightly lazy tongue that would sometimes get a little stuck when I spoke, but only I was aware of it. Gradually, my speech became more nasal and certain sounds disappeared altogether. The muscles of my lips, tongue and soft palate are weakening, and this greatly affects the formation of sounds that make words. Initially, the sounds that are made in the front of the mouth with my tongue and lips, like S, T, R, M, N, P and D, lost their sharpness or were absent from words altogether.

Dave likes to joke around. With my speech being difficult to understand, especially for people who don't spend a lot of time with me, Dave often has to translate what I say. This puts him in a position where he can basically say anything and pretend that I said it. The other day we had friends visiting from Cape Town. We were having dinner, and I asked something about their recent move to Cape Town. They couldn't quite make out what I had said, so Dave "very kindly" translated: "Jozanne says, 'Don't pick your teeth, John-it's rude.'" Needless to say, we all had a good laugh.

I can still communicate my needs effectively, but having a flowing conversation is becoming very difficult and tiring. Not only do I struggle with forming certain sounds, I also get breathless quickly. The muscles between my ribs and my diaphragm, which control the flow of air from my lungs through my vocal cords, have also weakened considerably, and I struggle to push the air out of my lungs. Speaking has become like running a marathon.

Recently, I was asked what had been the hardest part of this illness for me. That is not an easy question to answer, because my deterioration has taken place in stages and with each stage there has been something specific that has been difficult. When I first started using a wheelchair, I had to adapt to not being able to walk and run, but with the wheelchair I was still able to live a fairly "normal" life. Using a wheelchair didn't stop me from doing what I loved to do: interacting with family and friends. Then, when I couldn't use my arms and hands any more, it became more difficult, because I lost my independence, but at least I could still ask others to help me. At that stage the most challenging part was learning to receive and accept help from others. Dave and the children have been amazing in how they have been willing to help me, and of course my care-giver, Idie. But the children, especially, have made me very proud ... they never complain when asked to do something for me.

But the last six months have, by far, been the most difficult part of this illness that I have had to adapt to and will continue to adapt to. My ability to speak is my ability to interact with others personally. I am, obviously, still able to write with my computer and keep in contact with so many of my friends. I am very grateful for that, but there is something about one's voice that can say so much more than just words on a screen or page. What you say isn't always as important as how you say it. With your voice you can love, encourage, comfort, teach, and praise. With your voice you show your joy and your pain. People recognize you by the sound of your voice. They say that even before a baby is born, it learns to recognize its mother's voice and after birth it feels comforted just by the sound of her voice.

When I couldn't play with or hug my children anymore, I felt a great sense of loss and sadness, but I felt peace in knowing that with my words and voice I could still comfort and encourage them. To them, it didn't seem to make that much of a difference, they seemed to be content with the way things were. When they felt sad, I could still comfort them and, when they felt happy, I could still rejoice with them. But my voice has become flat and monotone. My words have become few and almost unrecognizable. Speaking has become hard work, not only for me, but also for those trying to listen to me. I know that the children understand the situation and that they don't feel neglected, but I know that they are not receiving a fraction of what I'm "giving" or feeling in my heart.

Luke is a sensitive and perceptive child. He can "read" me well and is able to anticipate a lot of what I am feeling. He likes to kiss and cuddle with me when he needs attention and will easily say how he is feeling. I can see he seems more secure in our relationship. Nicole, on the other hand, is happy and outgoing. She likes to perform and enjoys centre stage. Like all performers, she thrives on verbal encouragement and praise. When she needs attention, she likes to entertain me or be very animated in what she does, with the hope of an equally animated response. Sadly, I cannot give her what she needs anymore, and I can see that she is not feeling as secure in her relationship with me; but I know that even in this God is strengthening both of us.

I have, in the past, often taken speaking and communicating for granted, but it plays such a vital role in any relationship. I believe it is essential in a relationship. The better the communication between two people, the better or closer the relationship. I have come to learn that the same is true in our relationship with God. Prayer is vital and, just as our level of communication grows in a growing relationship, so also our prayer life should grow. For many years my prayers were like having a conversation with my boss: a bit formal and always putting my best foot forward, making sure to say the right thing at the right time. God felt distant and impersonal. I ended up praying more when things were going well, and when things were tough my prayers were few. I read in the Psalms how David prayed to God, and I longed for a relationship with the Lord like that. I thought I had a relationship with God, but I didn't really know how to rely on him. However, God is faithful and patient. When you draw near to him, he will draw near to you. "Come near to God and he will come near to you" (James 4:8 NIV).

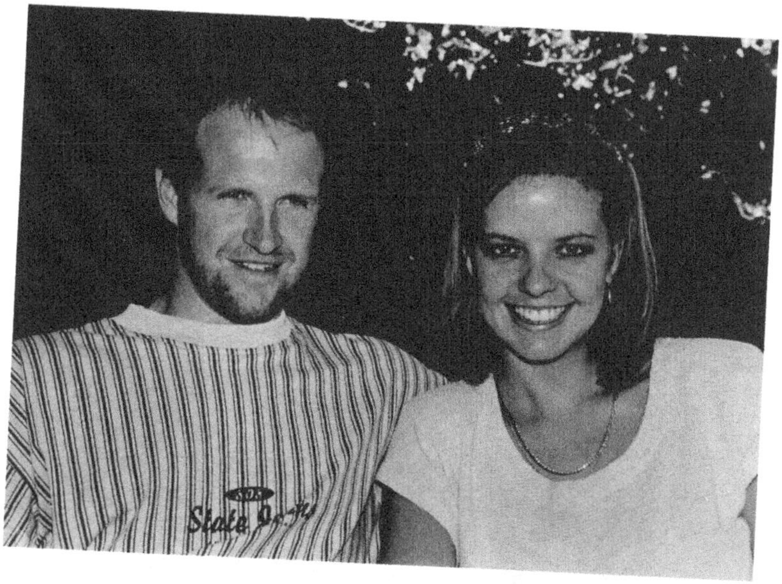

Dave and Jozanne started dating in 1994...

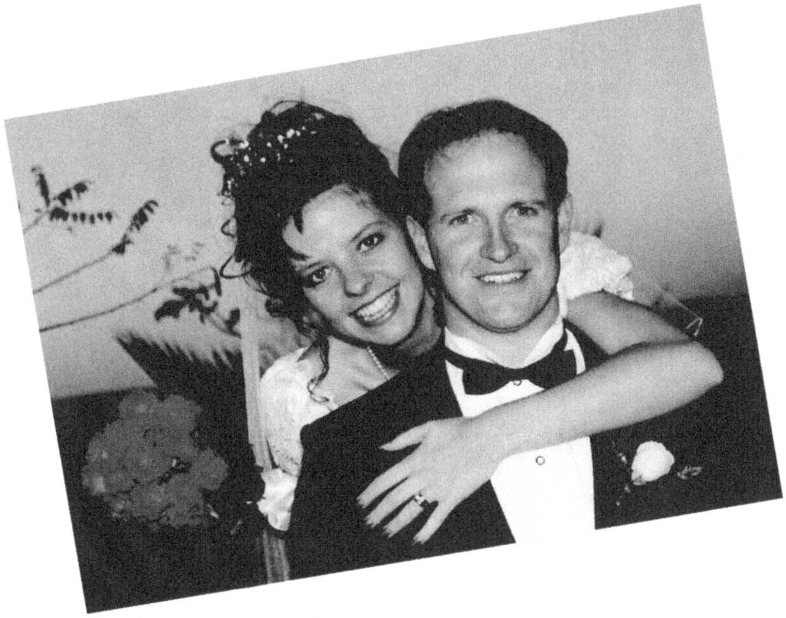

...and were married in 1995.

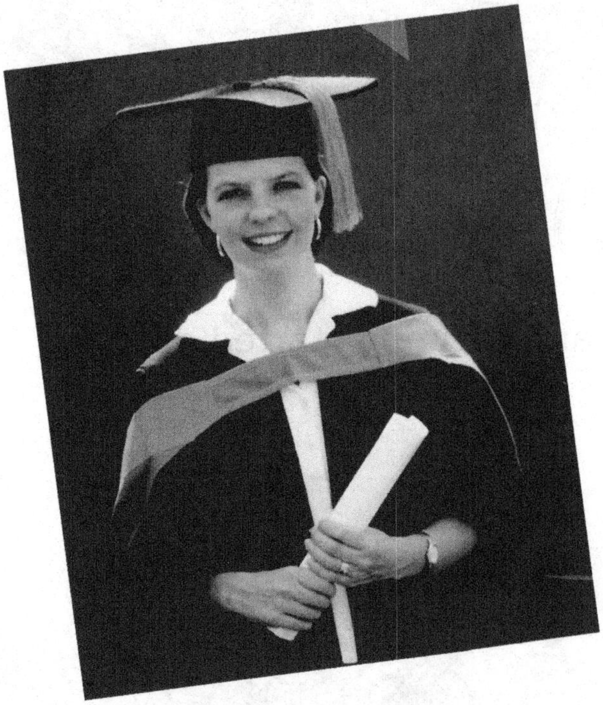

Jozanne graduating from the University of Pretoria in 1998 – BA (BPrimed).

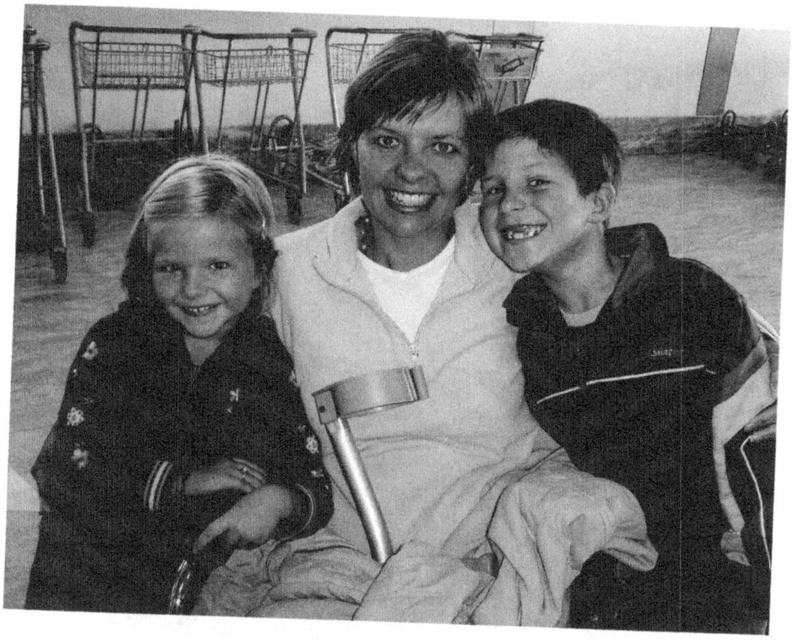

Shortly after hearing the diagnosis in 2005, Dave and Jozanne went on a trip to Europe. Here they say "Goodbye" to the children at the airport.

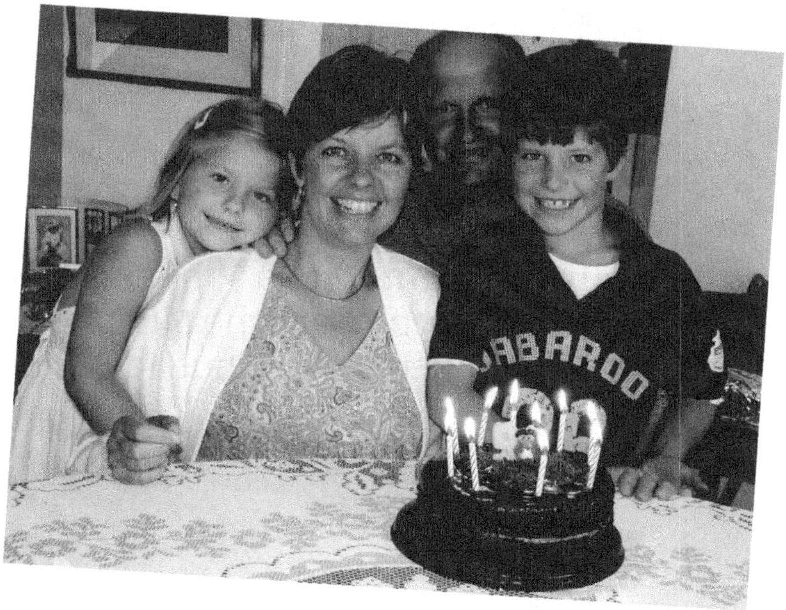

The Moss family celebrates Luke's 9th birthday in 2007.

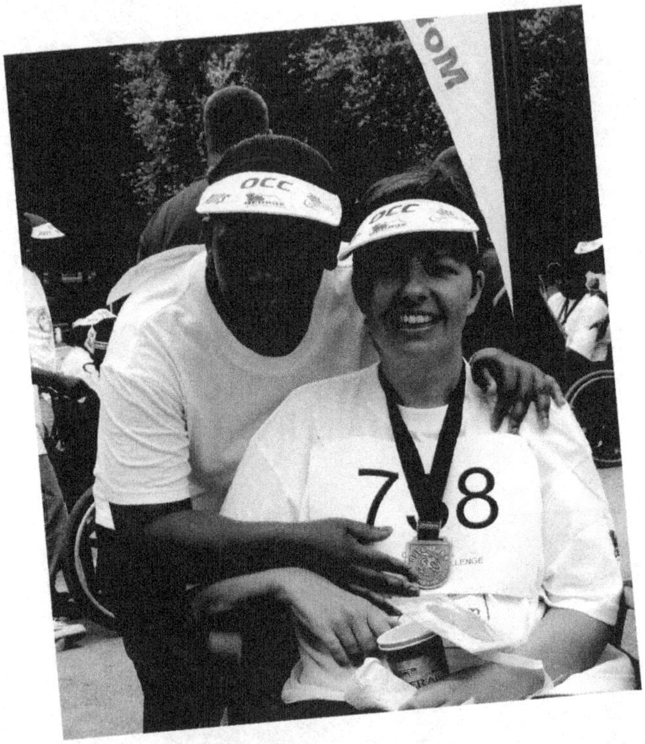

Jozanne and Idie after the Outeniqua Wheelchair Challenge, 2008. The family took part to represent the MNDA of South Africa. Jozanne comments: "I won the medal but Idie did the work!"

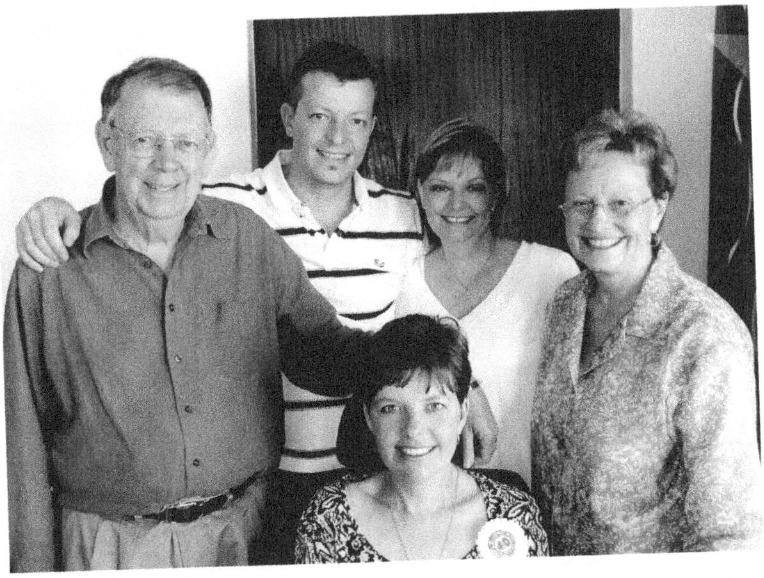

Jozanne with her family, celebrating her 40th birthday at Pinelake Marina, Sedgefield, in September 2008. From left, Kestell, Chris, Anna-Grett and Alma.

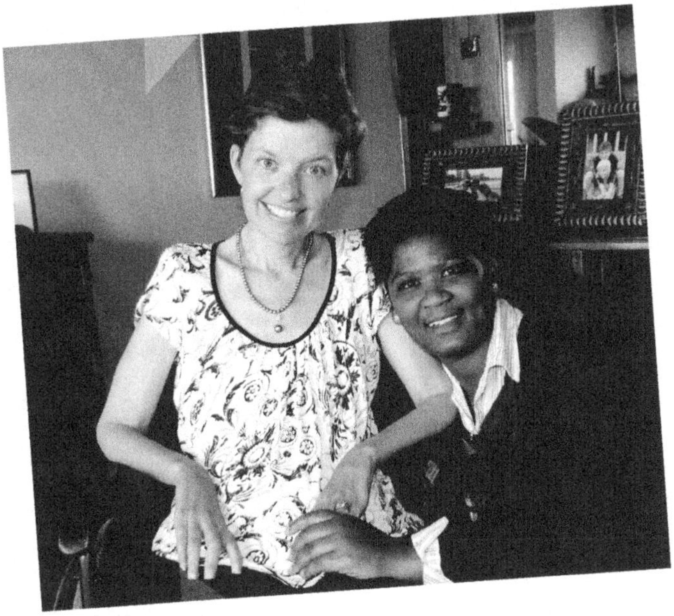

Jozanne with Idie ("caregiver and angel from God") in April 2010.

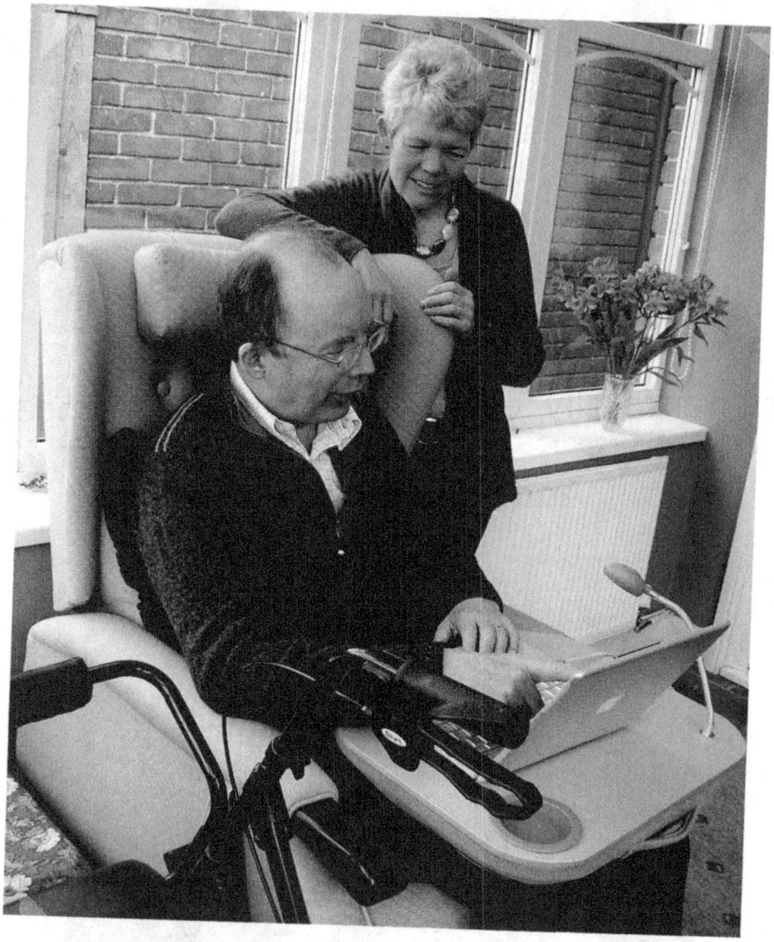

"At home" – Having now retired, Michael is dependent on Jane, his wife, and spends his time on his laptop writing and keeping in touch with friends on the Internet. (Bryan Wenham)

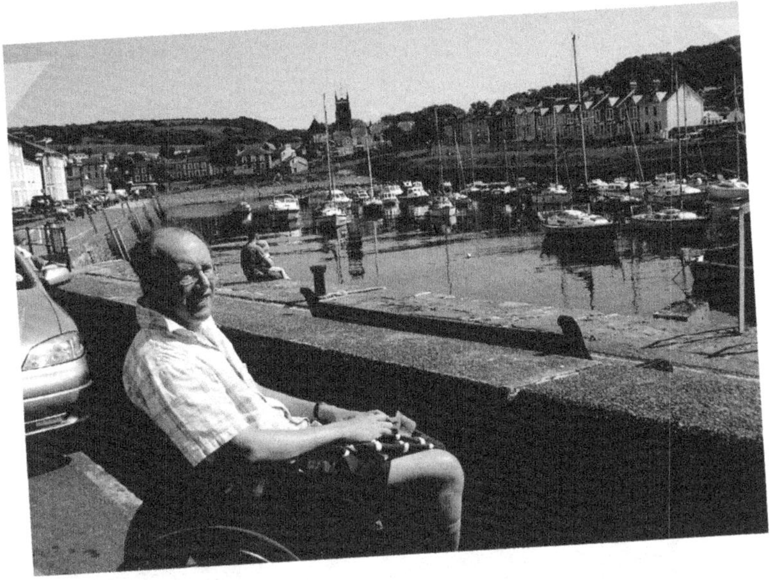

"Away" – Regular times away are important to break the routine of a prescribed life. While they can Michael and Jane have a number of bolt-holes, such as in mid-Wales. At Aberaeron. (Jane Wenham)

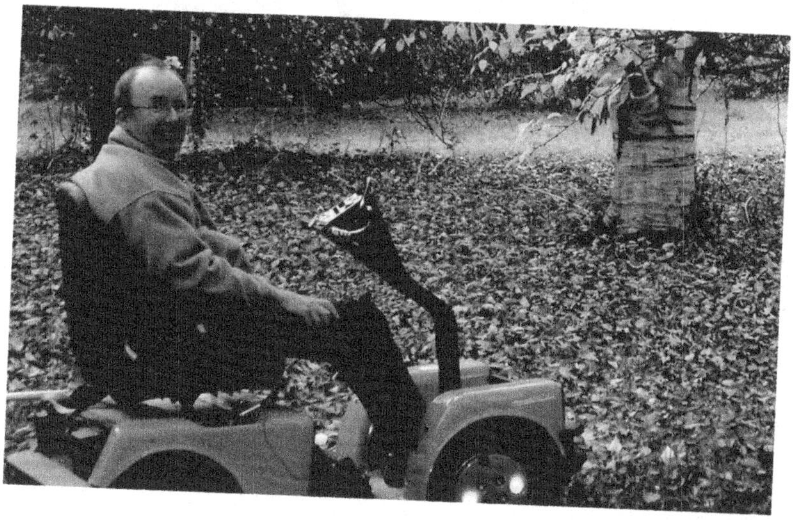

"Visits" – Days out are also a joy, especially when it's to somewhere you can borrow a powered buggy, as here at Barrington Court in Somerset. (Jane Wenham)

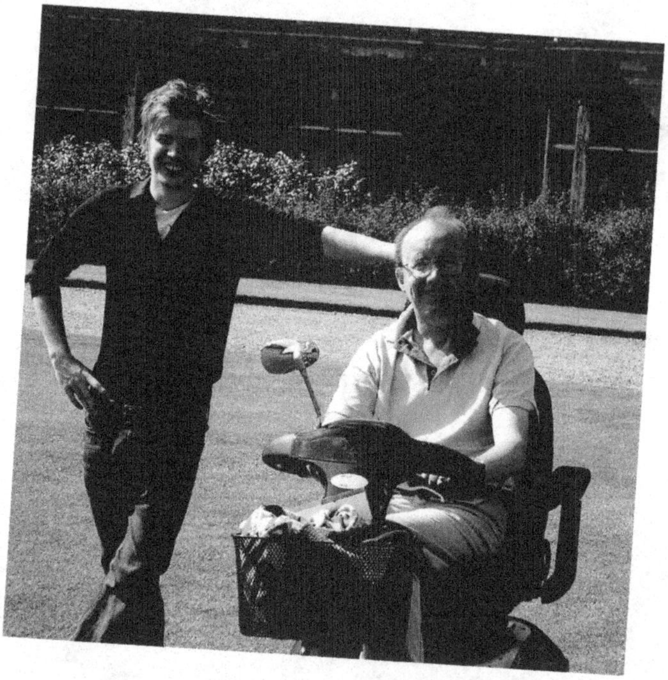

"Family time" – Holidays with the whole family have assumed a special significance in Michael's calendar. Here with youngest son, Bryan (and another buggy!) at Blickling Hall in Norfolk. (Jane Wenham)

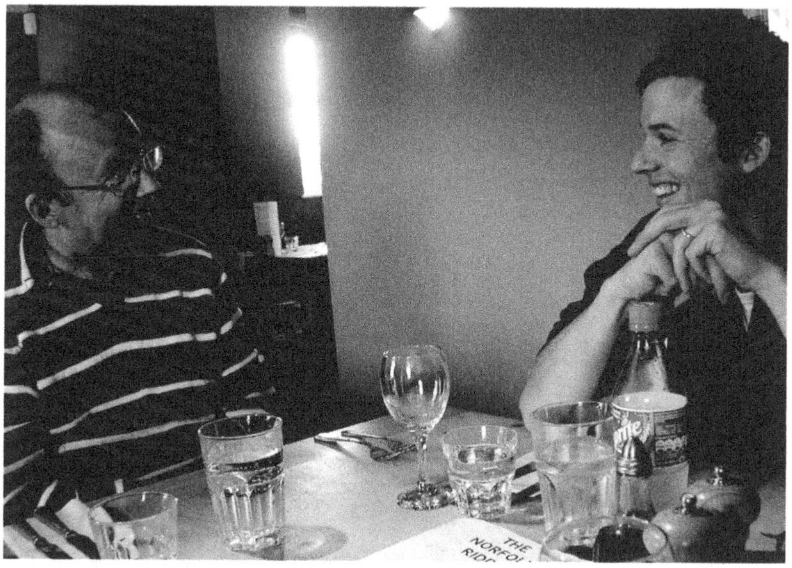

"Conversation" – Talking to family is treasured, here with oldest son, Paul. "We know it won't always be possible," Michael comments. (Stephen Wenham)

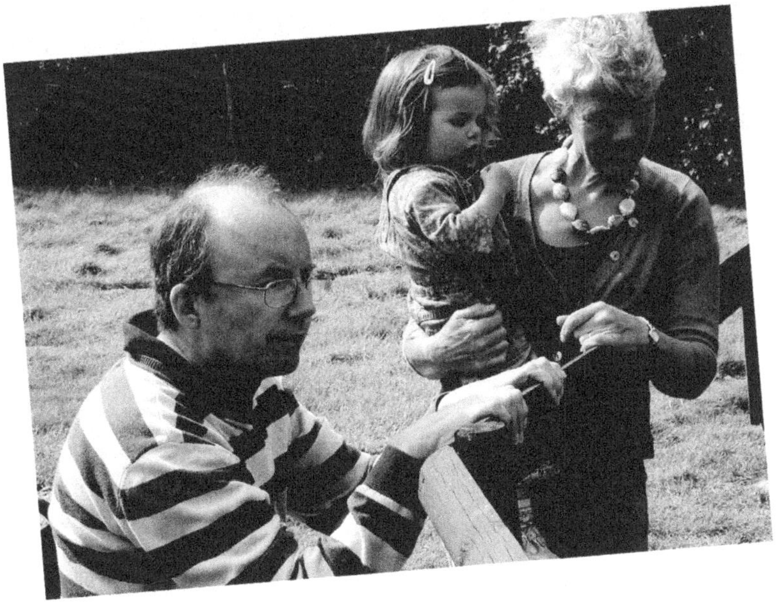

"Like a child" – It's still possible to share the wonder of discovery with their latest grandchild, aptly named Faith, in a small country park in Norfolk. (Rachel Wenham)

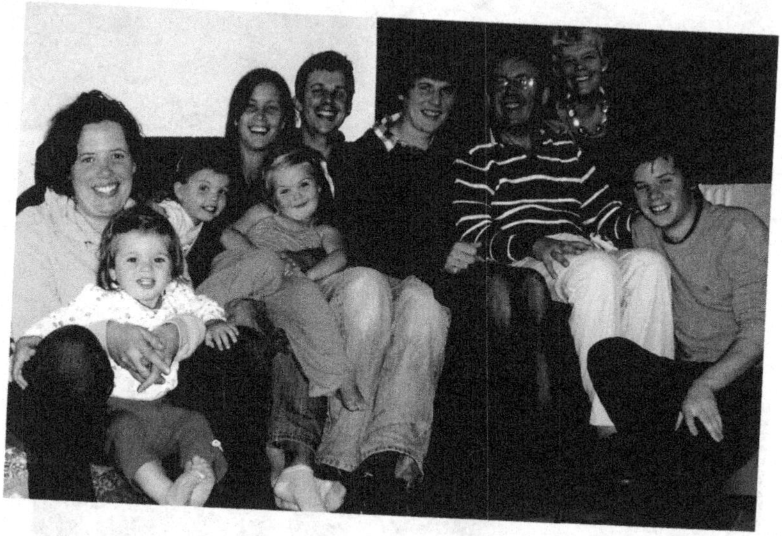

"I am blessed" – With the whole family, from right to left: Rachel, Faith, Lucy, Penny, Charis, Paul, Stephen, Michael, Jane, Bryan. (Bryan Wenham)

Through my illness God has stripped away everything that I could possibly turn to for security, those things that we don't realize we put our trust in. So often we think we are trusting the Lord, when actually our faith lies in our abilities, talents, and circumstances. I cannot *be* anything or *do* anything anymore. That may seem quite tragic to some people, but it has been such a privilege for me. It is so easy to get caught up in the things of the world, but I have nothing else to trust in. I have only God. He has shown me how to surrender completely – how to let go and let him. I feel free! I am in his hands; he is the driver and I am just along for the ride. I don't pray to my "boss" anymore; I pray to my Father, my Comforter, my Rock, and my Refuge.

God speaks to us so clearly through his word and we communicate with him through prayer. We have a living relationship with him and, just as we grow closer to each other by communicating more truthfully, so too we grow closer to the Father when we pray more truthfully. "Be joyful always; *pray continuallya;* give thanks in all circumstances, for this is God's will for you in Christ Jesus" (1 Thessalonians 5:16–18 NIV).

When God created us, it was with the purpose of having a relationship with us. Our sin separated us from him, but God had a plan for us to be reunited with him again. Through the blood of Jesus we can gain access to the Father again. What a privilege it is! My prayer for those who read this, is the prayer Paul prayed for his friends:

> *In him and through faith in him we may approach God with freedom and confidence ... For this reason I kneel before the Father, from whom his whole family in heaven and on earth derives its name. I pray that out of his glorious riches he may strengthen you with power through his Spirit in your inner being, so that Christ may dwell in your hearts through faith. And I pray that you, being rooted and established in love, may have power, together with all the saints, to grasp how wide and long and high and deep is the love of Christ, and to know this love that surpasses knowledge – that you may be filled to the measure of all the fullness of God.*

EPHESIANS 3:12, 14–19 NIV

CHAPTER 10

Praying truthfully

May your prayer of listening deepen enough to hear in the depths the laughter of God.

JOHN O'DONOHUE[20]

Having the power of articulate speech gradually removed affects all our relationships, including with God. Most effects are negative, but one is paradoxically positive. Something which Jozanne and I have in common, and probably share with ninety-nine per cent of believers, is a problem with prayer. For me, prayer tended to be a performance art; for her it was an interview with her boss.

As a vicar, almost the first casualty in my work was the praying of long liturgical prayers – which many regard as the glory of the Church of England. I used to take a pride in saying them clearly and making them comprehensible. I even understood the original meaning of "prevent" and "propitiation"! But then came the fall! My first symptom was my speaking, and at 8.30 in the morning a phrase like "a full,

20 John O'Donohue, To Bless the Space Between Us: A Book of Invocations and Blessings.

perfect and sufficient sacrifice, oblation and satisfaction" taxed my tongue and lungs to breaking point, while a word such as "institution" came out with half the letters missing. Why did the Prayer Book use so many Latinate words? It wasn't long before members of my congregation began helping me out, which was a blessing for them and a relief for me. This wasn't what T.S. Eliot meant by the "intolerable wrestle with words", though it began to feel like a fight. However, it soon became a struggle with meanings. Because much of my praying as well as preaching was *ex tempore* – as cynics might have said, off the cuff – as my ability to speak slowed me down and limited the words I could articulate clearly, I was afraid that my ability to lead worship would be limited. I certainly had to wrestle with simpler ways to express profound truths – and the result was probably none the worse for that!

I became, however, a man of fewer words. I had enjoyed conversation. I had relished debate. I admit it: I had fallen prey to the occupational hazard; I had grown to love the sound of my own voice! MND soon put an end to that, and as it has developed has made me much more taciturn. It's an effort to speak. It's frustrating that even my family, who know me best, even Jane, my wife, sometimes do not catch my meaning. It's not their fault. I just speak a cross between English and gobbledygook. And so I fall silent – and surly – which is unfair, and hard, on them.

This is something more than superficial, as it transfers to my personal prayer life. With God too, I am often silent and sulky. Yet, it has occurred to me that I am then being more genuine with God than I have been in the past, when prayers more often than not consisted of a string of requests with an occasional "Thank you" thrown in. It is what Jozanne calls "communicating truthfully", and is a component of real relationship.

It also allows God to get a word in edgeways, or perhaps for me to hear him, when my chatter has dried up. I have begun to believe that praying itself is more than a one-way conversation. Certainly, God speaks clearly to us through his word, the Bible, but not only this way. We don't know what the dynamic was in Jesus' own praying, but it clearly wasn't one-way traffic. Whole nights full of words to God? Hardly. How did he know the Father's will? When did he see what the Father was doing, or hear what he was saying? There is a great tradition of "waiting for the Lord" in his Scriptures, the Old Testament, summed up in Psalm 46:10, "Be still, and know that I am God." This is not an excuse for empty-headedness, a voiding of consciousness to make way for who knows what. It is a deliberate, even disciplined, attentiveness. Metropolitan Anthony of Sourozh describes it as "contemplation" which is "simply an attentive search through reflection, prayer, silence, and the deepening of the vision of things as God sees them. It has been said that prayer begins at the moment when God is the one who speaks. This is the goal towards which we must strive." Then he explains what specifically Christian contemplation is, because clearly anyone, even atheists, can attempt the search.

> *...the only difference is that the atheist observes phenomena, whereas we listen to the word of God who gives us the key to them. The difference seems small, yet everything hinges on it. For if we thus acquire the mind of Christ, if we are guided in the manner of the apostles (a manner that has not passed away with time), if we are guided by the Holy Spirit who enjoins us to go forth and act, to speak and to be silent, we are most certainly in the situation of the Christian.*[21]

In other words, effective Christian living begins not only on our knees but also in our listening at the same time. In the psalmist's words, "Let me hear what God the Lord will speak." (Psalm 85:8)

That, obviously, is not the whole story of prayer, as Jesus' answer to his disciples' request, "Lord, teach us to pray," and his other teaching on prayer indicate. There is clearly a place for intercession and praise and thanks. Yet, the first requests of the Lord's Prayer surely imply a prior listening to what the Father speaks, "Your kingdom come; your will be done on

---

21 Sermon: Prayer and Life © Copyright: Estate of Metropolitan Anthony of Sourozh, 1969.

earth..." Otherwise, they sound suspiciously like pious platitudes on our lips.

And how do you pray when you just don't feel like it? And what do you say when your heart is empty and you have nothing to say? These were questions which I faced with my lovely church family. They taught me that worship is a matter of the will, of intention. "Oh come ... Let us come into his presence ... Oh come, let us worship..." (Psalm 95) is an emphatic invitation, acknowledging human reluctance and continuing by hammering home how vital it is to "hear his voice" and have heartfelt engagement with God. "I will sing praise to your name, O Most High" (Psalm 9:2) is a declaration of intent. While we may well find ourselves echoing David, "I was glad when they said to me, 'Let us go to the house of the Lord!'" (Psalm 122:1). "I will" means more than "I am going to"; it means, "I want to and intend to, and I shall" rejoice, be glad. It can almost mean, "This may not be easy. I may have to grit my teeth, but I will do it."

But what shall I say? "How shall we sing the Lord's song in a foreign land?" (Psalm 137:4). What if all I want to do is complain and curse? One thing which is clear is that pretence is futile, with our God from whom no secrets are hidden. And so that psalm of bitter pain and alienation ends with possibly the blackest, most shocking verse in the Bible – which, if nothing else, encourages us to be honest. We have already seen the role of silence in prayer, which can apply in public as in private worship. But we still want to find words as well, because relationship works two ways. Jewish children probably learned all the psalms by heart; our book of Psalms would have been Jesus' prayer book – in his memory. Sometimes, as we know, he found the prayer he needed for the moment in one of the psalms. In the darkness of the cross, he begins to repeat Psalm 22. So for us, when our words strain and crack, we will find psalms to give expression to our inner thoughts. (That, by the way, is the reason for not just concentrating on our good old favourites and neglecting the less familiar psalms.)

Moreover, it is helpful to understand that the language of worship is the language of aspiration. In other words, sometimes, we will not feel that what we are saying or singing truly reflects our thoughts at the time. We may not feel on the one hand "miserable sinners", or on the other hand that God is "all I want ... all I've ever needed". And yet, we know both are profoundly true, and we would like to mean them. We aspire to mean them. In fact, of course, all worship is imperfect, just as all our knowledge now is partial; "for now we see in a mirror dimly, but then face to face" (1 Corinthians 13:12).

The final and magnificent resource we have been given in prayer is no less than the Holy Spirit of God, who bridges the gap between our feeble mortal bodies and the "throne of grace":

Likewise the Spirit helps us in our weakness.
For we do not know what to pray for as we ought,

but the Spirit himself intercedes for us with groanings too deep for words. And he who searches hearts knows what is the mind of the Spirit, because the Spirit intercedes for the saints according to the will of God.

ROMANS 8:26–27

I love that! It's as if our heartaches and longings which we can't articulate, or even identify, the Spirit knows and brings with perfect clarity and conformity to the Father's will into the Godhead – and creates the perfect prayer.

So ironically, as the disease has deepened Jozanne's prayer life and her relationship with her heavenly Father, so I have been taught basic and gracious lessons in prayer. I should have learned them long ago – and perhaps I did, though without such focus. However, that I should have been reminded of it now when my speech is failing me is a real gift of grace. After all, it is a common fear that, as our powers fail (including the "daughters of song" [Ecclesiastes 12:5]), so will our relationship with God. How good to know that it depends less on us, and increasingly, and in the end, entirely on him!

CHAPTER 11

Love at Jabbok

What, do you wish to know your Lord's meaning in this thing? Know it well, love was his meaning. Who reveals it to you? Love.

JULIAN OF NORWICH[22]

It was a particularly bad day – in fact it had been a bad week. We had been away for an October break to one of our favourite places. It was a real gift. The hedges and trees in the Blackmore Vale were at their autumn best: russets, yellows and greens. It had been a time to unwind after a busy year: retirement, moving house, settling in to a new environment and way of life – a roller-coaster of conflicting emotions, loss and bereavement, new beginnings, and excitement. Returning to a familiar place in a changed context emphasized the truth starkly. I wasn't working as a vicar now, and yet I seemed just as tired. There was no denying the tightening grip of the illness. And for the first time I wouldn't be going home to a situation where I had a role – even of minor sig-

---

22 A Book of Showings

nificance. I would be returning to be that anonymous character in the wheelchair, to be seen occasionally venturing around the alleyways of Grove, where we now lived. I had lost my identity, except in relation to Jane – and, when I saw them, my family. Moreover, I was assailed with the conviction that in the previous twenty years of my life the negatives far outweighed the positives. To put it bluntly, I had been a failure as a minister. It would have been better if I had never started. I understood the Preacher-King of Ecclesiastes in his dark moods: "What has a man from all the toil and striving of heart with which he toils beneath the sun? For all his days are full of sorrow, and his work is a vexation. Even in the night his heart does not rest. This also is vanity." (Ecclesiastes 2:22–23) And so, the week after we got back was a bad week, when reality kicked in.

It got worse. On a Saturday morning, as normal, Jane and I had our time of quiet and Bible reading. We had been reading from John's Gospel. The accompanying notes said:

> *The truth is that the whole point of Jesus' work on the cross is to make a way for us to know God (17:3). This isn't a casual relationship – we are welcomed into the family! Not only does God possess the power to do anything and everything he wishes, but he is also*

> *passionately interested in your prayers because he is passionately interested in you.*[23]

Somehow, I found it hard to say, "Amen", to that. Yes, I could have said it. But I didn't feel it, and I wasn't sure I believed it. The Creator of the universe is passionately interested in me? Jesus died on the cross for me? It was going to be a particularly bad day. I was not good company that day. And I wouldn't tell Jane why.

However, there was one part of that troubling note which unexpectedly proved true and significant: "we're welcomed into the family!" We did get to church on Sunday morning, where the pastor, out of the blue, had a word for "someone who believed they had failed, that they were a failure". He didn't know who it was, but God still wanted to use them. I listened! And then the next morning, we were having coffee with some new friends from the church. Talking about failure, she said very simply, "I think we all feel that from time to time, and you know, Michael, 'there is no condemnation for those who are in Christ'." Perhaps, I thought, God is interested in me after all. He may not be wielding his power to heal me, but he is aware of my thoughts. David was right:

> *O Lord, you have searched me and known me!*
> *You know when I sit down and when I rise up;*

---

23 Jonathan Bell in Closer to God, Scripture Union, November 2009.

you discern my thoughts from afar.
You search out my path and my lying down
and are acquainted with all my ways.
Even before a word is on my tongue,
behold, O Lord, you know it altogether.
You hem me in, behind and before,
and lay your hand upon me.
Such knowledge is too wonderful for me;
it is high; I cannot attain it.

PSALM 139:1–6

David's was a remarkable revelation indeed, as, whenever he worshipped in the Tabernacle, he had the constant symbol of God's otherness, the thick curtain dividing the Holy of Holies from the rest, behind which only the High Priest was allowed to venture once a year. God dwelt in unapproachable light.

I had a favourite video on YouTube. Max Kingston McCloghry was born at 12.05 in the afternoon of 27 February 2008. He died at 10.25 that evening. He was Matt and Jill McCloghry's first baby, born three months early. A week and a half later Jill was due to record a worship album for Hillsong Church in Sydney. It seemed an impossible ask: to sing worship songs with such a recent and raw grief. But she did, and the video was of her and her fellow vocalist, Brooke Fraser, introducing and then leading "Desert Song" in live worship.

This is my prayer in the desert
When all that's within me feels dry
This is my prayer in my hunger and need
My God is the God who provides.

This is my prayer in the fire
In weakness or trial or pain
There is a faith proved of more worth than gold
So refine me Lord through the flame.

I will bring praise, I will bring praise
No weapon formed against me shall remain
I will rejoice, I will declare
God is my victory and He is here

This is my prayer in the battle
When triumph is still on its way
I am a conqueror and co-heir with Christ
So firm on His promise I'll stand

All of my life in every season
You are still God
I have a reason to sing
I have a reason to worship

This is my prayer in the harvest
When favour and providence flow
I know I'm filled to be emptied again

The seed I received I will sow."[24]

Moving and defiant worship though the YouTube clip was (and I certainly couldn't have done it, even if I didn't croak like an old crow!), for me even more moving was reading the blog that Jill wrote that year. Its title is *{love}.* It is the record of a mother struggling with her grief and with God. It is her account of her journey through the desert, trying to sing the song in the fire and when the battle still rages, not just the song of words but the song of trust. It reminds me of Jacob wrestling all night with God at the stream of Jabbok as he returns with his family to the land of promise. Even when injured with a dislocated hip, Jacob will not let go of God. "But Jacob said, 'I will not let you go unless you bless me'" (Genesis 32:26). In the end, God blesses him with a new name, Israel ("He strives with God" or "God strives"). No longer is Jacob the deceiver. It is the name of the future;

---

24 Desert Song, words and music by Brooke Fraser © 2008 Hillsong/Thankyou Music/ASCAP (Admin. by EMI Christian Music Publishing and in the United States and Canada by Integrity Worship Music) c/o Integrity Media, Inc., 1000 Cody Road, Mobile, AL 36695. All Rights Reserved. International Copyright Secured. Used by permission. Reprinted by permission of Hal Leonard Corporation and Kingsway. Laura Hackett's Beautiful Mercy expresses the same experience in a more intimate style on her album 'Laura Hackett'.

his descendants will be called the children of Israel. And so he walks on with an eternal blessing and a lifelong limp.

For Jill McCloghry, her wrestling lasted not a night, but more than a year. And the wound-scar is still there. It's not possible to do her blog justice, but here are three extracts, which reveal the wrestling match between pain and faith, and the lifeline of God's love to which she clings.

25 June 2008

> Actually ... Some days I scream ... why us? Why the first child? Why can't You just fix this? Some days the most painful part of knowing the power of God is knowing that He in His might, could have fixed this in one moment ... but He chose not to.
>
> There is such a balance in this process of knowing that it is ok to question God ... to not understand ... to feel angry ... and on the other side of that to trust Him enough to rest in His sovereignty and know that He loves me more than any love I've ever known. To know that He knows my pain and carries it with me ... and to reverence Him and His power and trust that what He does is right and just and good. AHHH! I'm still working it out.
>
> This rollercoaster ... waking up ... crying ... worshipping and trusting ... crying ... feeling ok ... trusting ... crying ... being angry ... being

thankful ... missing Max ... crying ... sadness ... unexplainable joy.... it is absolutely what it looks ... a complete rollercoaster. But in this journey up and down and around again, I see the work of God. Showing me His beauty in the most unexpected of ways.

Yesterday, there was a knock at the door, and the delivery of the most beautiful flowers ... roses surrounded by flowers I had never even seen before ... the smell absolutely divine ... and a little note attached ... "We love you" ... from two of our best friends ... who while thousands of miles away had so thoughtfully and lovingly remembered that the week was Max's due date. These are the things that make my heart melt. The ways God reminds me that He has surrounded me with more love than I could have ever asked for. The best of friends. People that in the middle of their own busy lives know what pain our hearts feel and do something to show their love. I'm so thankful.

26 November 2008

Here's the thing.

The last week has been a rough one. I wake up in the mornings and feel the weight of the last year. I spend most of the day thinking about it. I think this is a week or so where I'm really beginning to process a lot of what's happened. Grief is a funny thing ... it comes in so many stages.

I sat on the bathroom floor weeping the other night saying to God – I can't take this anymore – I've had enough ... I really just hit a wall. The most amazing thing to me about having this relationship with God is that I CAN say those things to Him ... I can cry out ... grieve ... weep and He is there and I know that He is ever understanding and merciful ... and every stage of this is under His strong arm ... and even when I feel so far He is drawing me in close, tucking me under His wing.

I just felt like I should write today and say ... that no matter the feelings in your heart of grief or sorrow or the weight of your situation ... God is ok with you expressing these things to Him ... and the wrestling with Him, the questions, the unknown. He understands and is so merciful ... so good ... that He is walking all of it out with us. There is no instant fix ... not always a reason or rhyme, but there is grace ... and peace that surpasses all understanding ... that somehow shows up in the middle of a storm...

Today I feel like the disciples in the boat ... there's this huge storm raging all around ... waves crashing, thunder roaring ... and Jesus is a little bit silent ... sleeping ... but I just keep thinking.... I can't forget that one word in His time will quiet the storm ... quiet my heart ... still my soul ... and the word will come....

2 December 2008

9 months...

My little Max has been enjoying heaven for a few days over nine months now. I find myself thinking today ... what must it be like ... how amazing the sights he must see ... my son walking with Jesus knowing nothing but joy and peace, never feeling pain or sorrow.

Something about today, it resounds ... the greatness of God. He's protected Max from all the things in this world that could have hurt him or broken him. While I would give anything to love him in my arms, God has got that taken care of and I'm here loving him in my heart.

Max is knowing God deeper than I'll ever know him this side of heaven, and while I have my days of brokenness and confusion and hurt, God is doing so much more than I can see. He is truly weaving through Matty's and my life a cord of complete trust in our Saviour.

I've spent a lot of time in the past couple weeks with God trying to letting the pain and the things that are weighing on my heart be worked out by the One who created my heart. I'm still so very much in the middle of that process, but one thing I've learned so far ... nothing I've felt or experienced is out of His understanding or reach, no hurt too strong to scare Him away ...

> He sits with me, talks with me ... lets me say the things that I don't understand and He LOVES me.
>
> I love our Saviour. Jesus. Emmanuel. Holy Spirit ... Father. He is so good.[25]

I have no doubt that, in spite of her unanswered questions and experience of God's silence in the storm, Jill would be equally convinced as St Paul:

> *For I am sure that neither death nor life, nor angels nor rulers, nor things present nor things to come, nor powers, nor height nor depth, nor anything else in all creation, will be able to separate us from the love of God in Christ Jesus our Lord.*
>
> ROMANS 8:38–39

St John, in writing his Gospel, referred to himself as "the disciple whom Jesus loved". It's often misunderstood as a rather juvenile claim to being Jesus' favourite, or perhaps an unattractive arrogance. Actually, I am persuaded that this is a mistake; and that it should be read in something like an awed voice, meaning, "I've discovered that he loved this disciple, even me!" John is passionate about the love of God. It is the theme of his first and longest letter, summed up in "God is love" (1 John 4:8). "See what

---

25 Copyright © Jill McCloghry. Quoted by kind permission of the author.

kind of love the Father has given to us, that we should be called children of God; and so we are" (1 John 3:1). You could translate the final four words: "And that it is what we are!" Jesus used different analogies to express God's love for us: lost children; friends, not servants; and one which the poet George Herbert focused on in his poem, "Love". One by one, God (Love) overrules the excuses of the guest to the great banquet. From beginning to end it is all grace, smiling grace full of love, welcoming us not to wait at table or to wash up, but as honoured guests, to be served by *him.*

Love bade me welcome; yet my soul drew back,
Guilty of dust and sin.
But quick-eyed Love, observing me grow slack
From my first entrance in,
Drew nearer to me, sweetly questioning
If I lack'd anything.

"A guest," I answer'd, "worthy to be here:"
Love said, "You shall be he."
"I, the unkind, ungrateful? Ah, my dear,
I cannot look on Thee."
Love took my hand and smiling did reply,
"Who made the eyes but I?"

"Truth, Lord; but I have marr'd them: let my shame
Go where it doth deserve."

"And know you not," says Love, "Who bore the blame?"
"My dear, then I will serve."
"You must sit down," says Love, "and taste my meat."
So I did sit and eat.

The picture is of someone invited to a meal, and arriving at the door dirty and shabby, and realizing he is in no fit state to come in, but his host will have none of it because it seems he really wants him. In the last verse, did you notice, it shifts from being an account of a conversation between Love and the soul in the past to including the present? It's as if Love is addressing us as well. He *says,* "Don't you know that I took the blame for you?". "He himself bore our sins in his body on the tree" (1 Peter 2:24). Our stock, and rather religious response, is to *do* something, to "serve". The guest wants to help, to justify his being there, "Let me give you a hand in the kitchen!" But Jesus didn't die in order to make us servants. "No way!" Incredibly, he wants us as friends sharing his meal with him, enjoying his company (a word originally meaning "sharing bread" together): "You must sit down, and taste my meat." The poet tells us his response, but leaves us to make ours.

I love Holy Communion, or whatever name you give it, the Mass, Eucharist, or the Lord's Supper. At the very heart of the service, sinners – betrayers, deniers, and deserters – all are invited to come, and we come with empty hands to receive the gifts of the One who is Love. *The Lord Jesus on the night when he was betrayed took bread, and when he had given thanks, he broke it, and said,*

> *"This is my body which is for you. Do this in remembrance of me." In the same way also he took the cup, after supper, saying, "This cup is the new covenant in my blood. Do this, as often as you drink it, in remembrance of me." For as often as you eat this bread and drink the cup, you proclaim the Lord's death until he comes.*

1 CORINTHIANS 11:23–26

As the hymn "Rock of Ages" puts it: "Nothing in my hand I bring/Simply to Thy cross I cling". Grasping God's love for us personally is essential when we are faced with a test on our faith, and the cross is the crux of that love. In a different but profound way, Jozanne has come to understand and experience that same Love in her illness.

CHAPTER 12

A mother's love

Can a mother's tender care
Cease towards the child she bare?

WILLIAM COWPER[26]

Jozanne's Story

The most amazing thing that has happened to me in my life has been becoming a mother. I have probably learned the most about God's love for me through becoming a parent myself. Back in 2005, when I was diagnosed with Motor Neurone Disease, I immediately felt peace in my heart about dying. I wasn't afraid. I was shocked, but I wasn't afraid. I knew that after death I would be with God in heaven. Obviously, many things went through my mind at the time, but fear for myself wasn't one of them. I felt complete peace. After a few days, when the shock had settled, the sadness started. I felt sad about many things, but the saddest thing was the emotional pain that lay ahead for my children.

---

26 Lovest thou me?, Olney Hymns, 1779

Dave and I became part of a Motor Neurone Support Group that gets together once a month for a meeting, and a great time to laugh with and chat to others who are in the same situation as we are. About ten people attend these meetings regularly, of whom four of us have MND. With every meeting we usually have a guest speaker to address an area of need like a physiotherapist, speech therapist, neurologist, dietician, and so on. These meetings are of great value to us. They allow you to gain important information from the specialist, but also from other patients, and to hear how they deal with the various difficulties we have to face daily. At our most recent meeting, our guest speaker was a doctor who specializes in palliative care. She works at the hospice in George where they take care of terminally ill patients in their last stages of life. She discussed death with us, and the various care options that are available. She also discussed the role of counselling for the patient and also for the rest of the family. For example, counselling for preparing children for the death of a parent. As you can imagine, this was a very difficult meeting.

A mother's strongest instinct is to care for and protect her children. I remember with both my kids, when they were babies, like all mothers, I would deprive myself of many things to ensure that my babies were comfortable and happy. Their needs always came above my own. When they started crawling and then walking, I did everything I could to keep them from hurting themselves – from rearranging furniture, to jumping up in a split second to put my hand over the sharp corner of an object so that the inevitable bump of a head would be painless. And when, at times, I couldn't prevent an accident from happening, I would be just as sad as my child.

When Luke was almost three years old, I received a call from his playschool one day to say he had fallen, hitting his mouth on the edge of a table. They said he seemed OK, but that he wouldn't stop crying and probably only needed his mommy. I rushed over right away and was shocked to see his little T-shirt covered in blood from the neck down. The teacher showed me the cut in his lip and said it would heal quickly; but I wanted to be sure; so I took him to the emergency room. When the doctor pulled his lip open, his one front tooth fell out. I was shocked. The root of the tooth had to be surgically removed the following day, and Luke was left with a very painful mouth and fat swollen lip. I don't know who was more traumatized, Luke or me! But it was a horrible experience for both of us. I felt so helpless, and wished I could take the pain away for him, but I couldn't. Today, obviously he is fine and can't even remember any of it. (I remember it like it was yesterday.)

For Christmas 2006, we gave the kids a big, round trampoline. We had thought the decision through carefully because of the dangers involved and decided that, with a good set of rules, the kids should be fine. All went well, and the kids had loads of fun during the December holidays. We remained consistent with our safety rules. In January 2007, Nicole started grade 1. She was so excited and loved everything about school. On the last weekend of January we allowed the kids to go on a church picnic with friends. I couldn't help wondering, every now and again, whether the kids were being looked after properly, especially on the trampoline at the picnic spot. I felt relieved when they returned home safely at about 5p.m. They had enjoyed themselves very much and told me all about their day as I lay on my bed. Minutes later, Nicole went outside to play on the trampoline ... To my horror, I heard a shriek that will probably stay with me for ever. The shriek was followed by silence, and, as I called Dave, Nicole came running with her left arm bending backwards just above the elbow.

It was a terrible fracture that needed surgery a week later. They had to put two steel pins in her arm to stabilize the shifted bones. This was followed by two weeks off school, the arm in a cast for two months and follow-up surgery, almost a year later, to remove the pins – not to mention all the pain and suffering she had to go through. It was all so traumatic. Was there anything I could have done differently? I wish I could have taken her pain away, but I couldn't. Today, of course, she is perfectly fine. In fact, she has grown into a tough young girl who loves all things outdoors and sporty.

It is sometimes so painful to be a mother. We worry so much about our children and try so hard to protect them:

"Who are they driving with to the hockey match?"

"Hope they're wearing seat belts."

"I don't want him to be teased at school."

"I'm scared the hockey ball hits her in the face."

"Why won't the fever break?"... Yet, we really have very little control over what happens to them. We have to let them live their lives. We have to let go and allow them to learn, even though it is painful at times. We can only trust God.

I say this confidently, but it is probably the hardest thing I have ever had to do. It seems easier to trust God with myself and my life, but my kids are a different story. I know my death is going to cause them terrible pain and there is nothing I can do to prevent it. I cannot soften the blow. I cannot fully prepare them for what lies ahead. I cannot minimize the pain even slightly. I can only trust God – and I do, but with a deep sadness. In this sadness I hold on to God's word. "And we know that in *all* things God works for the *good* of those who love him, who have been called according to his purpose" (Romans 8:28 NIV).

But what is my job then as a mother? Is it to be there for them, driving them to all their sports and activities? Is it to help them with their homework and assignments? Is it my job to make sure they eat healthy food and get a good night's sleep? Or, to teach them not to put their elbows on the table, or to speak with a mouth full of food? Is it my job to nurse them when they are sick, and to kiss it all better? Or, to bake delicious cookies and to arrange special birthday parties? Yes, it is; but that's not all! I know as parents it is our job to teach our children good manners and respect for others; to teach them life skills and social skills, discipline and self-respect. It is our job to provide them with a home and to make them feel safe and secure. It is our job to prepare them for the future as best we can ... But even if I could do all these things to the best of my ability, I still could not protect them from the consequences of living in a broken world:

> *Therefore, just as sin entered the world through one man, and death through sin, and in this way death came to all men, because all sinned.*
>
> ROMANS 5:12 NIV

> *We know that the whole creation has been groaning as in the pains of childbirth right up to the present time.*
>
> ROMANS 8:22 NIV

The biggest and most important thing I can do for my children is to teach them about God's amazing love for them and Christ's saving grace. I can prepare them by teaching them about eternity and about their purpose here in this life. I cannot shield them from pain and suffering, but I can teach them who to turn to and where to find their strength. It is in our suffering that we grow.

> *Therefore, since we have been justified through faith, we have peace with God through our Lord Jesus Christ, through whom we have gained access by faith into this grace in which we now stand. And we rejoice in the hope of the glory of God. Not only so, but we also rejoice in our sufferings, because we know that suffering produces perseverance; perseverance, character; and character, hope. And hope does not disappoint us, because God has poured out his love into our hearts by the Holy Spirit, whom he has given us.*
>
> ROMANS 5:1–5 NIV

CHAPTER 13

In the mirror

In all the setbacks of your life as a believer God is plotting for your joy.

JOHN PIPER

Jozanne's Story

Can you imagine what life would be like if there were no mirrors? Most of us use mirrors on a daily basis, or at least most women. I can't speak for men, but, when I observe my husband, I am convinced that many men also need mirrors daily, even though they won't admit it. How people behave in front of mirrors is where the differences between men and women are evident – or are our similarities then evident?

From a very young age, my daughter, Nicole, has been fascinated with mirrors. I have the most beautiful photos of her at the age of three, looking at herself as she dances in front of a full-length mirror. She loved the movement of her body and enjoyed watching these various movements in the mirror. Even today, she loves to perform in front of the mirror. She is forever trying out weird and wonderful hairstyles or creating new fashions with different items of clothing. Many facial expressions, with the voices to match, are also tried and tested, repeatedly. I am convinced she was born a true performer. Now that she is able to do her own hair for school, it is astounding to watch the whole procedure that plays out in front of the mirror in the morning.

My son, Luke, on the other hand, is a different story. I have photos of him as a baby, noticing his reflection in a mirror and all he was interested in was to play with the other baby in the mirror – or at least, to taste him! Even now, Luke really hardly ever looks in a mirror. In the morning before school, we have to remind him to comb his hair. He really could not be bothered. When he does eventually look in the mirror, it doesn't seem to make much of a difference. He still manages to miss most of the hair on his head. I know this is a "boy thing", which won't last for much longer. Before we know it, Luke will be a teenager and then, I am sure, the mirror will become very important to him.

Have you ever watched men lifting weights in the gym? That section of the gym is usually surrounded by mirrors from wall to wall. The bodybuilders parade around looking at their bulging muscles, but that is what the sport is all about. They have a specific way of flexing their muscles when they look at themselves in the mirror. My husband, Dave, is not a bodybuilder but sometimes, when he doesn't know I am watching, he also likes to flex his muscles in the mirror. I am sure most men are like that, but, as I mentioned earlier, this is where men and women are probably more alike than different. Yes, women are probably the biggest culprits when it comes to admiring themselves in the mirror. I should know because I am one.

I won't say I have been obsessed with mirrors but, like many women, I have sometimes allowed my happiness or mood to be determined by what I see reflected back at me in the mirror. There have been many times that I have allowed how I look to determine how I feel. Now obviously a person needs to take pride in how they look. You need to be clean and neat, not sloppy and unkempt; but what I am talking about goes beyond that. As women, we know what it is like to have a "bad hair day"; no matter what you do, your hair just won't do what it is supposed to do. Unfortunately, we often allow this to affect how we feel about ourselves and inevitably how we behave. Or, you feel you have gained some weight and when you see yourself in the mirror, your confidence drops to the floor. You see yourself for what you look like and not who you are.

There is another side to this scenario, when things are actually not going well at all and we may be very unhappy, but to hide this fact, we dress ourselves up, put on make-up and do our hair. Then we look in the mirror, put a smile on our faces and go out into the world and pretend we are fine. I have been guilty of that too. I think it started in my teens and continued far into adulthood. As I have matured, not only emotionally but also spiritually, my confidence has also matured. I have grown to accept who I am and how God has made me, and that I am unique. However, once again God is calling me higher.

Like cancer and many other devastating illnesses, MND is a ruthless disease. Although it is a disease that affects the nervous system, it inevitably affects the body. You eventually lose the function of all your motor muscles (voluntary muscles). When a muscle is not used it starts to shrink, just like when the plaster cast is removed after a broken arm or leg has healed. The healed limb is usually thinner, but recovers after normal use of the muscle resumes. This shrinking of the muscle is called atrophy. One of the telltale signs that my doctor noticed when my diagnosis was made, was the atrophy of my left thumb muscle. That part of the hand that looks a bit like a chicken drumstick had shrunk, like someone had eaten all the meat off the drumstick. Obviously, my left hand had also weakened.

In the first two or three years of this illness, I didn't really notice any more muscle atrophy taking place apart from in my hands. In fact, to my dismay, I even gained some weight because of my inactivity from being in a wheelchair. But in the last year, or even six months, without any effort, I have lost about 18 kilograms. Under normal circumstances I would be overjoyed! I had finally reached that dream goal weight, that "golden" number that I probably last weighed in high school and that I had always dreamed of weighing again. My clothes are hanging loose on me and it's such a great feeling. I have even had to buy smaller pants because my pants are falling down, and I don't even walk. I emailed my sister in Australia just to brag about my new weight. We had both dreamed of weighing this much for years.

A few weeks ago I asked Idie, my care-giver, to help me to stand in front of a mirror so that I could take a look at this new slimmer me. Because I am in the wheelchair, I never get to see myself in the mirror beyond my shoulders. I was quite excited, and even embarrassed that I was prepared to go to such great lengths to see myself in the mirror. That morning, after my regular shower, instead of getting dressed immediately, Idie with much effort, lifted me up from my wheelchair and balanced me in front of a large mirror. It took me a few seconds to register what I was seeing in the mirror. It wasn't what I expected. It is one thing to lose fat while toning your muscles, but that's not what I saw. In the past six months I had lost 18 kilograms of muscle. My shoulders, elbows and knees look big and bony, and my hip bones stick forward. My skin seems thin and loose. My arms and legs have no muscle to give them any shape. My stomach muscles are non-existent and so my tummy pushes out. I was shocked!

The reflection I saw in the mirror was not a person I knew. I felt sad. Motor Neurone Disease had now finally taken hold of my whole body. However, just as God has been there to encourage me in all the previous phases of this journey, he once again encourages me with the wisdom and truth of his word.

Therefore we do not lose heart. Though outwardly we are wasting away, yet inwardly we are being renewed day by day. For our light and momentary troubles are achieving for us an eternal glory that far outweighs them all. So we fix our eyes not on what is seen, but on what is unseen. For what is seen is temporary, but what is unseen is eternal.

2 CORINTHIANS 4:16–18 NIV

The person I see in the mirror may not be a person I remember, but the person on the inside is also different. She is faithful, hopeful, and free. She is a new creation and her life has purpose. I wouldn't exchange that for anything.

Praise be to the God and Father of our Lord Jesus Christ! In his great mercy he has given us new birth into a living hope through the resurrection of Jesus Christ from the dead, and into an inheritance that can never perish, spoil or fade – kept in heaven for you, who through faith are shielded by God's power until the coming of the salvation that is ready to be revealed in the last time. In this you greatly rejoice, though now for a little while you may have had to suffer grief in all kinds of trials. These have come so that your faith – of greater worth than gold, which perishes even though refined by fire – may be proved genuine and may result in praise, glory and honour when Jesus Christ is revealed.

1 PETER 1:3–9 NIV

CHAPTER 14

Worship in the wilderness

We've become so used to the idea that suffering is to be avoided at all costs, that the very notion that we might have to bear it is seen as a violation of some emerging right to a minimum level of comfort. But suffering has a positive purpose.

M.R. HALL

The idea that there could possibly be any positive purpose in suffering is an alien concept in societies where risk and discomfort are assiduously avoided, and insured against. After all, pain relief is a great blessing. Biting on a block of wood while having one's leg sawn off is unimaginable. Thank God for anaesthetics, and antibiotics, and even airbags! Everyone agrees. The person who dares to suggest that suffering might in some sense be positive is howled down as inhumane, as indeed the novelist M.R. Hall was, when he wrote an article in *The Guardian* newspaper headlined, "Life is sacred – don't downgrade it" (29 January 2010). I will return to the main theme of his article, which was assisted suicide, in the next chapter. He sees the positive mainly in its potential for good in those who care for the sufferer, and its vital part in creating a society which truly respects life. Of course, he admits, it's tough and not fair on the sufferer. But both Jozanne and I would say that it's not entirely true. Indeed, Jozanne's remarkable testimony has already made that clear.

Finding meaning in suffering

> *Thus says the LORD, the God of Israel, "Let my people go, that they may hold a feast to me in the wilderness."*
>
> EXODUS 5:1

I had never noticed the second half of the verse before. I suppose I kept hearing the magnificent voice of Paul Robeson singing *Let my people go:* "Go down, Moses, way down in Egypt's land, tell ole Pharaoh, to let my people go." I think I assumed that either it was a pretext to escape slavery (as Pharaoh probably did!), or that they had just had a party to celebrate getting out. However, I now think there is something more profound going on.

God is summoning his people into the wilderness in order to worship him there. We sometimes entertain the illusion that the desert wanderings of the Hebrews were a sort of prolonged picnic with sandwiches laid on each morning and barbecues every evening. That, of course, is far from the truth. The Sinai and Negev deserts are far from hospitable places – freezing at night, baking in the midday sun. Unprotected, it doesn't take long to suffer from dehydration and heat exhaustion, which quite soon proves fatal, as one of my sons almost discovered ... The wilderness is harsh – and wild. It's certainly not comfortable. Yet, it's here God wants to be worshipped. Not waiting until they reach the "promised land", the land flowing with milk and honey, where they will be able to settle and build a monumental temple, but in the testing conditions of the desert. Why?

What's special about the desert? The desert plays a formative role in the spiritual lives of a number of heroes of faith in the Bible from Jacob, Moses, David and Elijah in the Old Testament to Paul in the New. For Jesus himself, it is where his ministry is forged both negatively in the temptations and positively in angels refreshing him. "And Jesus returned in the power of the Spirit to Galilee," Luke concludes (4:14). Far from being the place where God is not, the desert seems to be where he calls and meets his people.

In the unique and somewhat strange love story of Hosea, there is a verse which has been especially important to me for the past two years:

Therefore, behold, I will allure her,
and bring her into the wilderness,
and speak tenderly to her.

HOSEA 2:14

The prophecy of Hosea is addressed to God's faithless people, "Israel", who are committing "adultery" with idols, and is God's appeal to win them back by all means. He wants to bring her back to her first love. However, the message is for us too. We are the people whom God loves – the discovery that John made, as we noted. He loves and he woos us. And the wilderness is where God speaks tenderly to us. Many, if not most of us, are so tied up with the encumbrances of our comfortable lives, that to be honest, listening to the whisper of the divine Lover, the "still, small voice", is impossible. And yet he is longing to communicate his love to us, to tell us he loves us, in order to restore the original covenant, that first love relationship that we have let go cool. What an incredible truth – that the desert experience can be the time when we meet his love, again! But it should not, perhaps, surprise us, for the moment of supreme love for us was the moment of his supreme desolation in the darkness.

I am *not* for a moment saying that God inflicts wilderness times on us in order to bring us to our senses, or somehow to force us to love him. But I am not the first to suggest that God invites us to meet him in the desert. What I am saying is that he is there when it hurts and when it's dark and when you feel you can't take anymore. We have already quoted Psalm 139 7–8:

Where shall I go from your Spirit?
Or where shall I flee from your presence?
If I ascend to heaven, you are there!

If I make my bed in Sheol, you are there!

There is nowhere that God is absent, not even illness and death. I am saying he can speak tenderly to us when we are in the depths.

Not so long ago, I was asked that direct question: "Where has God been in your experience of MND?" and I gave the "right answer", but knew that wasn't enough. I needed to be more specific. Where had I actually met him? Where had I actually heard him? Where exactly had I experienced his love?

So I began to make a list:

- unconditional love of my family
- faithfulness of friends
- kindness of "strangers"
- professionals' care & MND Association's concern
- unlooked for provision and perfect timing
- moments of beauty and time to enjoy them
- moments of truth, particularly when the Bible has "spoken" to me
- Holy Communion, when I receive the tangible tokens of his sacrificial love.

It clearly is not an exhaustive list, but is sufficient evidence of God's presence. The first six one might describe as God's love reflected on to me from different mirrors; the last two as more direct whispers of love, but all of them are signs of God's love for me.

If only I will see them. We have a choice whether to meet God in the desert or not. It's very easy to be so body-bound and so wrapped up in the struggle for survival – as I am, I confess, often – that we don't even want to meet him. It's as if he is in front of us, but we are just looking at the ground. Near the end of her harrowing and intensely moving book about her unborn daughter, Cerian, *The Shaming of the Strong,* recounting an utterly wilderness experience, Sarah Williams writes:

> *Everyone hurts. At some stage most people find that life does not deliver what we expect it would or should, and sometimes, worse still, life damages us directly. Although we may use our strength to control what happens to us, often we have little power to prevent difficult things happening. What we do have, however, is the power to choose how we respond. Everyone can choose to turn towards God and to love him, in spite of the difficulty and injustice, even in the midst of a situation ... All we would have without him, is the illusory freedom of our own strength to protect ourselves and our autonomy to isolate ourselves.*[27]

We know that God is there, in the desert. We know that he is love and for that reason is always looking for the creatures he loves. But love "does not insist on its own way". That is why it must be our choice to meet God; he's already made his choice. It seems to me our choice in his direction is our worship in the

---

27 Sarah Williams, The Shaming of the Strong, The Challenge of an Unborn Life; Life Journey, Eastbourne, 2005, page 171.

wilderness, our "desert song", as Brooke Fraser has it. At times it can be little more than the decision to lift our face towards him, or to hold one of those hand-shaped holding crosses, or the silent breathing of his name, in response to what Laura Hackett calls his "Beautiful Mercy".[28]

In 1984, Professor Frances Young wrote a book entitled *Face to Face* "with assistance from Arthur", who was her eldest and disabled son, aged seven. It was revised and republished in 1990 with the sub-title: "A Narrative Essay in the Theology of Suffering", which gives a good idea of the original, relating the pains of having and bringing up a severely disabled child in the late twentieth century – and the pains could be unbearable. Thus, there are successive chapters called "Face to Face with Doubt" and then "Face to Face with God". In the midst of her desperate doubts, she has two remarkable encounters with God, which bring her joy and peace. God has met her in the desert. The book begins with her Psalm of Testimony, of which these are some verses:

I will exalt you, O Lord,
for you have drawn me up from the depths,
and have not suffered hopelessness to
triumph over me.

---

28 In her album Laura Hackett MP3 (International House of Prayer, Kansas

O Lord my God, I cried out in my emptiness,
and you have made me whole...

...the Lord drove me into the wilderness
and hid his face from me.

Vainly I cried out, What is your will, O God?

The Lord afflicted me,
he made me taste the waters of bitterness,
creation's sadness;
my first-born was handicapped...

As I journeyed on my way,
again he spoke to me:

Go, teach and preach,
be my minister.

For this I prepared you from birth,
for this I led you through the wilderness,
for this I am setting you on your feet
and putting my joy and love
within your heart.

Then my heart leapt within me,
and my being was filled with song:

O give thanks to the Lord for he is good,

for his mercy endures for ever...[29]

God is there in the desert. In the desert he speaks tenderly to us. We will worship him, for he is good. His steadfast love endures for ever.

29 Frances Young, Face to Face, © Frances M. Young 1985, Epworth Press, London, pages 3–5.

CHAPTER 15

Just for laughs!

The greatest happiness of life is the conviction that we are loved, loved for ourselves, or rather loved in spite of ourselves.

VICTOR HUGO

Jozanne's Story

I have shed many tears since my diagnosis with MND, but many of them have been tears of laughter. Laughter is a wonderful thing ... They say laughter releases "feel good" hormones in your brain that can actually make you live longer. All I know is that laughter is good, was created by God and can be found in any situation – although not always appropriate, I suppose. But I think having a good sense of humour helps to make even the toughest situations seem easier.

When God allowed this illness to come my way, he gave me everything I needed to be an "overcomer". He gave me hope; he increased my faith, and he also increased my sense of humour. He taught me how to laugh at myself, and at, as well as with, others in situations that might not seem to warrant laughter, but where you have to just laugh, otherwise you might end up crying – and, let's face it, laughing is much more fun.

The most amusing part of my illness has been the many different ways in which people have reacted and responded to the changes that have taken place, at various stages of my illness. *My comments are by no means meant to hurt or insult anyone, because I know I would have reacted in exactly the same way.* I am merely amazed and amused by our "human nature", and how society has taught us to respond to illness, disability, and even death. I am sure, at times, the Father must laugh at our humanness. The most refreshing responses I have experienced have been from children, because of their honesty and realness. This helps me to understand why God tells us to be like little children in order to see the kingdom of heaven.

In 2005 I was teaching grade 1 at a primary school in George. By about June or July of that year, I started experiencing the first symptoms of my illness, a lazy left foot that I had to lift a little higher than the other in order to walk without tripping. Initially, the kids in my class didn't notice anything different. But by November, when the diagnosis was made, my unusual, clumsy walk was evident to all. The school year ended with its usual hint of sadness, after being with a class for a whole year, and then having to pass them on to a new teacher. I also decided to stop teaching then.

By March of 2006, I started using a single crutch to assist my walking and to help with balance. I used a normal crutch, the kind that has a part for your hand to push onto, with an extended section that supports your elbow. One Saturday morning, I was at the shopping mall with my family, when I bumped into one of the kids I had taught in the previous year. The wonderful thing about teaching young children is the amount of love and affection you receive from them. When this child saw me, she immediately ran to me with open arms to give me a big hug. The crutch got in the way and made the hug a little uncomfortable, but that didn't seem to worry her much. "Mrs Moss!" she exclaimed with a big smile. "Look, Mommy. It's Mrs Moss." She then stepped back and took a good look at the crutch on my arm. With a puzzled look she asked, "What's wrong with your *arm,* Mrs Moss?" I just had to laugh.

On another occasion, not too long after, I was at the movie theatre with a friend and we were standing in the queue to buy popcorn. By now, my balance had deteriorated a little more, and I had to concentrate more to remain steady on my feet. The crutch now became like an anchor when I stood still. Suddenly, out of the crowd, almost from behind, a little girl from my Sunday school class ran up and gave me a huge hug around my legs. As you can imagine the force and momentum was too much for me, and the two of us started to topple over, almost in slow motion. Fortunately, the rest of the queue behind me broke our fall and no injuries were sustained. Then, in one swoop, the highly embarrassed father of the little girl picks her off me, and in the same motion gives her a smack on the bottom. At the same instant, many hands in the crowd lifted me up, and within seconds I was back on my feet. All the attention is on "the poor lady with the crutch", but all I can think of is the poor little girl, whose frightened face disappeared into the crowd as quickly as it had appeared. *She* needed the attention and concern, not me. I am the adult; she is the child.

For many years, Dave and I dreamed of taking a trip to Europe one day. Our plan was to wait for the day when we would have some extra cash and time on our hands – as if that day would ever come! So as soon as we heard of my diagnosis and the progression of the illness, we decided not to wait any longer. In May 2006, we left for a three-week tour of Europe. We chose, as part of our trip, to go on an organized bus tour, which travels through eight countries in twelve days. Realizing that the trip would be very busy and tiring, we were advised to take a wheelchair with us. I was walking with the aid of the crutch and, although I was still managing to move around confidently, I walked much more slowly and tired more quickly. The wheelchair would be there as a backup, in cases where we might have to cover long distances on foot. I ended up having to use it only three times. I guess if someone had told me that one day I would need a wheelchair, the streets of Rome, Florence, and Amsterdam would not have entered my mind. But God is good, and he has encouraged and carried me on every step of my physical deterioration.

The trip was wonderful. In Florence, we had an afternoon where we could just walk around and explore at leisure, and so we took the wheelchair. When one is able to walk, you are in the driver's seat. You decide where you want to go – right? Obviously! Who even thinks about that? But this all changes when you are in a wheelchair. You become the passenger; and that takes some getting used to. We ended up in a beautiful town square with various coffee shops, and many, many gift and souvenir kiosks. This was the ideal opportunity to buy things for family and friends – or so *I* thought. This became the first of many lessons in surrender that, I am sad to say, I failed. There were just too many different things to see and directions to go in, and poor Dave could just not keep up with his demanding "back seat" driver. We were both tired and ended up having a fight. Dave decided to go his way, and I decided to go mine. So, I got up out of the wheelchair and started pushing it – to the amazement of people sitting at the street cafés, who witnessed the "miracle".

By January 2007, I was no longer able to walk without putting myself and others in danger. Although I still had the strength in my legs, I did not have the balance or coordination to be able to walk. That's the thing with MND: the nerves that send the messages "to move" to your muscles from your brain and spinal cord, just start dying off, and you are unable to use those muscles. I suppose it was at this point that I officially qualified as a physically disabled person. I even received my official wheelchair tag for the car. This opened a whole new world to parking possibilities. Going to the shopping mall on a Saturday morning now became a completely stress-free experience, as far as parking is concerned. (Just one of the perks of being disabled!)

Having previously been an able-bodied person, I remember walking in a busy shopping mall with hundreds of people rushing past one another, all preoccupied with the 101 things that they needed to do. The people around you were just a sea of faces and you hardly ever made eye contact with anyone. But my experience of this changed completely in a wheelchair. Becoming a "passenger" instead of a "driver" now gave me the opportunity to observe others more. What became apparent was that when you are in a wheelchair you don't blend into the sea of faces anymore. People notice you. I remember in the beginning I was more aware of it. People would often respond in one of two ways. Some would be walking along with their straight, focused faces until they spotted me, at which point their faces would turn to what Dave and I like to call the "cheesecake" smile (shame, "the poor lady in the wheelchair" smile). There is another group of people in this crowd who would behave in a very different way. They also spotted the lady in the wheelchair from a distance, but then would go to great lengths to look the other way, almost turning their necks off.

Then there are the children. When they see a wheelchair, especially the younger kids, they stare long and hard, and some even ask: "What's wrong with your legs? Why can't you walk?" Distressed and embarrassed parents would immediately grab their children away, and sometimes even apologize. What for? I don't know! I just love their honesty and openness, and I love chatting to them. I am sure many adults wish they could just ask: "What's wrong with you?" We grown-ups can make things so complicated!

Another thing I have noticed since I have been in a wheelchair is how some people speak to you. They bend forward and speak more slowly and loudly, making sure to pronounce each word clearly: "H-o-w/a-r-e/y-o-u?" I know they mean well; but I do have a chuckle every now and again. I have also noticed how some people would rather speak to whoever is pushing the chair than to me. Once, when I went shopping with my friend Tara, we approached a shop assistant and I asked her about a product I was looking for. She responded, but only looked at my friend and asked her, "What type is she looking for?" I replied, but the lady seemed to avoid making contact with me. I think fear makes people behave strangely. I will have to try not to be so scary in future!

More recently, my speech has deteriorated quite a lot. I struggle to form certain letters like S, M, P, D, T, and, in Afrikaans, the "G" sound. Words come out muffled, nasal, and hard to understand. *I* now have to speak slowly and clearly; so I don't blame people for thinking I have a hearing problem. But with this new phase in my illness, I am confronted with a whole new range of comical experiences. Like I have said, you have to laugh at life and human nature. The other day I bumped into someone I hadn't seen for some time, and she asked me how I was. "I'm fine, thanks. It's just that my speech has deteriorated quite a lot," I said with difficulty. I thought she might not have understood me when I saw the look of panic on her face. She responded with, "Oh, that's very nice!" and an uncomfortable smile on her face. I had to laugh to myself. I get the feeling that people think they will offend you, if they ask you to repeat yourself when they haven't heard you clearly. (Do they think I don't know that my speech is poor?)

In March, it was my son's birthday and he had a swimming party. As the party drew to a close, the parents started arriving one by one to fetch their children. I was familiar with most of the moms, but I had not met many of the dads. One of the dads who arrived came over to introduce himself. He reached out his hand to shake mine, not knowing that I couldn't lift my hand. After a few uncomfortable seconds, he realized the problem and handled the situation very well. He then continued to ask me how the party had been, and I proceeded to answer his question. I shouldn't laugh, but the poor man had no idea what he had let himself in for. He could not understand a word I was saying (and I don't blame him). Nervously, he started looking around to see if anyone could rescue him. Someone did. Another mom came over to say "Hi", and the dad saw his opportunity to disappear.

We humans are strange creatures when faced with unknown situations. We try to pretend that we are in control, when in fact we often have no idea how to respond. We try so hard to keep up appearances, instead of being real and honest. I guess human nature is exactly what it says: "human" nature, not "God's" nature.

CHAPTER 16

Family and friends

Walking with a friend in the dark is better than walking alone in the light.

HELEN KELLER

Jozanne's Story

My frame was not hidden from you when I was made in the secret place. When I was woven together in the depths of the earth, your eyes saw my unformed body. All the days ordained for me were written in your book before one of them came to be.

PSALM 139:15–16 NIV

Even before we are born, God knows us, and he determines where we will live and who we will be born to. He chooses our parents and our families. We don't have much of a say in the matter – or perhaps I should I say, they don't have much of a say. On the other hand, we do get to choose our friends, or rather, they get to choose us. As we go through the various phases of life, often our circle of friends also changes. Some friends stay for a lifetime, while most enter our lives for a period of time, only to leave again as our roads part. But with family it is different, they stay part of your life whether they want to or not.

As a schoolgirl, I never really had many friends. There was always just one special friend, but, because I went to four different primary schools, even these friendships were not that close. High school wasn't any different: I only had one real friend, but within the first year after school we lost contact. As a student at university, I lived at home and didn't really get very involved in student life on campus. This was purely by choice and, although I longed for an existing student life, I lacked the confidence and self-assurance to be a friend to anyone. Only once I started working, and after I became a Christian, did I really start building true friendships. I know this became possible, because of a newly found confidence. For the first time I could be myself and feel accepted, not because of who I was, but because of who Christ is.

As I look back at my life now, I can divide my friendships into two main groups: before the diagnosis of my illness and after the diagnosis. The "before" friends, can further be split into those who are still around, and those who are not. Because we relocated to George shortly before I became ill, not many of the "before" friends are still around, but a number of them have made a lot of effort to keep in contact with us, and support us, and for that I am very grateful. There are some who are able to visit us whenever they get the chance, and there are so many who continually pray for us. I don't really have the words to truly express how much I appreciate these loyal and loving friends from the "past". I do know that they mean more to me than they realize, and that God is using them to encourage and inspire me as I travel on this difficult journey.

The second group of friends that I referred to, the "after" friends, are a very special group of people. What makes them so special is the fact that they have chosen to be a part of my life at this very difficult time when, in a worldly sense, there is very little I can offer in return in terms of friendship. As I have said, in the eyes of the world, I am not a good friend to have, but by God's grace, I am part of a body of friends who love and serve me with God's love.

> *The body is a unit, though it is made up of many parts; and though all its parts are many, they form one body. So it is with Christ.*
>
> 1 CORINTHIANS 12:12 NIV

> *If one part suffers, every part suffers with it; if one part is honoured, every part rejoices with it. Now you are the body of Christ, and each one of you is a part of it.*
>
> 1 CORINTHIANS 12:26–27 NIV

Amazingly, God has placed each friend in my life for a specific purpose, according to the gifts he has blessed them with. I have friends who pop in from time to time with words of encouragement, or with a hearty meal for the family. I have other friends, who have taken over some of my motherly duties with the kids, by carting them around to and from school, sports, and other activities. I have friends who look after my spiritual well-being and love me enough to tell me the truth, even when it hurts. And then I have friends who have come alongside me, to walk this road with me, on a more daily basis. For all of them, I am eternally grateful because of the sacrifices they are making. My prayer is that God will bless them with the measure that they have blessed my life. Each of these friends are important to me, and make my life richer.

But now, for the most important and most special people in my life, my family. They did not choose to be on this journey with me; they were chosen. When Dave and I were married, almost fifteen years ago, he promised to love me "in sickness and in health". All married couples promise that; but I think very few really count the cost of what it means, when they say "I do". I know I didn't give it much thought at the time, but, when Dave said "I do", he meant it. The last four years have not been easy. In fact, life has become exceedingly challenging as time has passed, but Dave has, in all aspects, stayed true to his promise. In many ways, this journey is much harder for him than for me. Not only has he lost the wife he once had; he has had to take over a lot more responsibility, and has had to carry the family on his own, but he is also the one I take my frustrations out on when things get too tough for me. Yet, he perseveres and continues to love me with an unfailing love. I am facing death and the *certainty* of heaven, but he is facing loss and the *uncertainty* of raising two children on his own. I love and appreciate him very much.

My children are also on this challenging journey with me without any choice or free will, but they have been true warriors. Although our situation may seem sad and tragic to the world, we do not live in that sadness on a daily basis. My kids are normal kids, and we have a "normal" family life. There are rules and boundaries like any other family. There is praise, and there is also punishment where it is due. The kids sometimes take chances as all other kids do. Some days they think we are "cool" parents, and other days they don't. This is the only family life they know; so why would they feel that they are missing out on something? All families do things differently, and so do we. The advantage for my children is that they are learning, from a young age, that some people have special needs, and that life is not always easy, but that with God we can overcome anything. My kids are sensitive to the world around them, and they appreciate what they have. They are strong and loving, and very special to me. I love them very much and wish they didn't have to suffer the pain of loss one day, but I know that God loves them even more than I do.

The rest of my family are very special too. My mom lives in George, very near us. Like Dave and the kids, she is also part of this challenging and painful journey, not by choice but by blood. My father is also close by, but he has escaped the reality of life. He suffers from Alzheimer's disease, and is unaware of the world around him. I wonder sometimes – is that a good thing, or a bad thing? I miss him very much. Sadly, my mom is faced with two very difficult situations, but she is a strong woman – much more than she realizes – and even in her pain God has a perfect plan. I love and appreciate her very much.

My two siblings fall into a whole other group, the "past/present" group. They both live far away, and only get to visit maybe once a year. They know me from the "past" but don't really share the "present" with me, although I know they wish they could be here more often. Because of the deteriorating nature of this illness, every time they visit, I think, they get a bit of a shock and have to adjust their minds to the new reality. People who are around me regularly, don't experience my deterioration so radically, and are obviously not as distressed when they see me. My sister, Anna-Grett, and her family have just visited from Australia. She was here about a year ago, but I hadn't seen her husband, Jon, and sons, Kyle and Craig, in about three years. It was so special to see them all again, but I couldn't help feeling sad to imagine their shock and pain. This is also a situation that they did not choose to be a part of, and yet, I know they love and support me, and I am very grateful for that. I love them very much.

As I look at all the people whom God has surrounded me with, friends and especially family, I feel blessed and so loved. I experience God's love for me, through them. God's plan and purpose is always perfect. If love were a currency, I would be a very wealthy woman.

CHAPTER 17

The Power in weakness

Give yourself fully to God. He will use you to accomplish great things on the condition that you believe much more in His love than in your own weakness.

MOTHER TERESA OF CALCUTTA

Jozanne's Story

Within days of my diagnosis, I had peace in knowing that God had a plan and a purpose with my life and my illness. I didn't just hope it or believe it. I knew it. There is a peace that comes with knowing. I didn't know what the plan was or how God was going to use me, but I had no doubt that he was going to use me – and that it was going to be good. This knowing comes from God. If I think back, it was quite a challenging time for me spiritually, because I felt a certain sense of expectation to put God's plan into motion. This expectation was not placed on me by God, but by myself.

I was very eager to be used by God, but I had not yet learned what true surrender was. I was still very focused on what I could and should do. At the same time, I was trying to deal with the reality of facing a terminal illness, even though my only symptom was this lazy foot. Being told I was dying just didn't seem real. It really was a confusing time for the whole family. While Dave and I were trying to deal with the shock of this new reality, and with the difficulty of telling family and friends, we were also trying to protect the children from the truth and maintain a sense of normality at home. So, one minute I would feel devastated, especially when we would share the news with others and see their reaction. The next minute I would feel almost excited, knowing that something big lay ahead for us, but uncertain what. It was extremely difficult for me to share this with anyone, including Dave. God gave me the peace and I couldn't make others feel it too. This, I know now, was my first lesson in surrender and trusting God.

The first year or two seemed a bit of a blur for me, but I know now that God was preparing me for what lay ahead. I didn't always see that, and was often caught up in fighting the physical battle with a body that was gradually becoming weaker and more stubborn. The physical changes and challenges were becoming more and more obvious, but I was unaware of the spiritual changes that God was making in preparation for his purposes. There were times when I felt overcome by the situation. But then God would encourage me with his wisdom and insights, spoken to me through his word, devoted friends and even my children. While I was weakening physically, God was strengthening me spiritually. Through my physical battles, I was learning spiritual lessons about his love for me, and how to put my trust in him.

As time went by, I started reading books about other people with illnesses and struggles, and how they dealt with and overcame their circumstances. This made me think that maybe God's plan for me was to write a book about my life story, to inspire others. When Sandy, a good friend of mine, also suggested I write a book, I eagerly jumped in and started writing. At that stage, I could still type but with some difficulty. It seemed like a mammoth task ahead of me. Where do I begin? Do I start with my conversion or the diagnosis? Do I write about my childhood, or only my adult life? What about my life would inspire others? These were some of the questions I struggled with. I started several different chapters, and when typing became difficult I dictated my words on a tape recorder, and then my friend would diligently type everything for me. Eventually, even speaking and recording became difficult, and I stopped. To be honest, I wasn't very inspired by what I wrote and wondered how anyone else would be inspired. I was trying so hard, but it wasn't working. I wasn't a writer.

In the meantime, a few Bible study groups had invited me to share my testimony with their members. It was a great honour for me to share with others how God had given me so much peace, despite my circumstances, and how he had surrounded me with such love. This inspired people – not me and my story, but him and his glory. Maybe this was God's plan with my life and my illness. Maybe I was meant to speak to groups of people. It brought me a lot of joy to speak to these groups, and the way people responded to God's love really encouraged me. Again, God showed me that he was in control, not me, and I finally felt that God was using my life for his glory.

As time went by, my speech started becoming more and more unclear. I knew the illness was running its course, and prayed along with friends, that God would save my speech for as long as possible, so that I could fulfil his purpose for my life. I must admit that at times, I felt disappointed that it was all coming to an end so soon, but I was grateful that, for a time, God could use me to make a difference in others' lives. What a privilege!

But I am still learning that God's thoughts are so much higher than ours. Someone very kindly donated a laptop computer to me, for the purpose of communication when I lost my speech completely, eventually. With modern technology I was once again able to type using one finger, a mouse and an on-screen keyboard. So when I was again invited to speak to a group, I decided to type what I wanted to share about "healing", and then asked Dave to read it. Afterwards, a few people asked for copies of what I had written and asked whether they could share it with others. I was so encouraged by God's new plan.

I decided to revisit the chapters I had written previously, with the hope of maybe finding new inspiration to complete what I had already started. I also tried other topics like writing about life, death, joy, and suffering. I tried very hard, but I was never quite happy with what I wrote. I felt that I was trying to be an expert in areas that I knew nothing about and again I gave it up. This was obviously not how God was going to use me. I also realized that I was trying too hard to do what I thought God wanted me to do, and while I was learning to surrender physically to my situation, God was teaching me how to surrender to his will spiritually. I decided to stop trying and to start trusting.

One day Dave asked me what the things were that I missed the most in my life, and that I wished for. I couldn't answer him immediately, because I hadn't really allowed myself to dwell on thoughts like that. So I gave it some thought, and decided to make a wish list. I wished for many things that I could no longer do, and the list seemed quite sad, but by the end of the list, God showed me that only one thing really mattered, and that was the wish that my kids would one day also know the love of God. I emailed my wish list to Dave and a handful of friends. They were encouraged by it and shared it with others, and that is how God began his ministry in me. I started writing down what God was teaching me in my situation. If God inspired me through it, I knew he would inspire and teach others with it.

I now send my emails to over a hundred people around the world, who also forward them to their friends. I have met so many people on the Internet, and received many replies from people who have been encouraged and inspired by what God is teaching them through my life. I feel so privileged and honoured to be used by God in this very special way. God is making full use of modern technology, and has even enabled a DVD to be made of our family, describing God's goodness in our difficult circumstances. Part of it has been put on YouTube, where God can reach many, many more people than I could ever have imagined. This has all happened in the last six months.

> *Now to him who is able to do immeasurably more than all we ask or imagine, according to his power that is at work within us, to him be glory in the church and in Christ Jesus throughout all generations, for ever and ever! Amen.*

EPHESIANS 3:20–21 NIV

The last six months have shown the most and fastest period of deterioration in my illness. I have lost a lot of weight, my breathing has become more strained, my speech has become almost inaudible, and I have become a lot weaker, but God has used me more in six months than in the forty-one years that I have been alive. I have never felt as happy and fulfilled as I do right now. I might be weak, but with God I am strong. I might seem powerless in the eyes of the world, but through me flows the power of God.

Three times I pleaded with the Lord to take it away from me. But he said to me, "My grace is sufficient for you, for my power is made perfect in weakness." Therefore, I will boast all the more gladly about my weaknesses, so that Christ's power may rest on me. That is why, for Christ's sake, I delight in weaknesses, in insults, in hardships, in persecutions, in difficulties. For when I am weak, then I am strong.

2 CORINTHIANS 12:8–10 NIV

CHAPTER 18

Give me joy

God, you have made us for yourself, and our heart is restless till it finds its rest in you.

AUGUSTINE OF HIPPO[30]

Jozanne's Story

At the birth of a new baby, parents wait anxiously for the cry of their newborn child. This cry fills the parents' hearts with joy because it is a sign of life and health, a screaming newborn is usually a healthy baby with strong lungs. It is funny though, that the parents spend the next year or two of their lives going to great lengths to get their baby to stop crying. The most wonderful feeling for any parent is when this new little person that has entered your life makes eye contact with you and gives you a big smile. Parents will do strange things to make their baby smile and giggle with pleasure, from pulling weird faces to making strange sounds, all for the joy of seeing their little one happy.

---

30 Confessions, Book 1, Chapter 1 (translated from the Latin by Michael Wenham.)

It doesn't take a lot to make a child happy. I remember with both my kids wanting to make sure that they were sufficiently stimulated with the best educational toys for their age, only to find them having more fun with the inside of a toilet roll, and the lid of a can of deodorant spray. It is only as they grow older that it has become a bit more difficult to impress them. I don't have teenagers yet, but from what I hear it takes a lot as parents to make them happy, if at all. But one thing is sure: everyone wants to see those they love happy – although, I think, as parents we sometimes try too hard to make our children happy, and end up doing more harm than good.

For many years I searched for joy and happiness, as I am sure everyone does, but I never quite seemed to find it. I knew true joy and happiness were out there; I just had to find them. I obviously had happy moments and periods of time, but who can possibly be happy all the time? I remember being in primary school and thinking that once I was in high school, then I would be happy. Then I would be a little older, and people wouldn't treat me like a child anymore, I thought. But then in high school I remember thinking that probably once I left school and became an adult in charge of my own life, only then would I really be happy. Well, I left high school, went to university, found a boyfriend and even earned extra money doing student work at a local restaurant, and still something was missing. Although people and situations made me happy on the outside, deep inside me there was still an emptiness that left me feeling discontented and unhappy. Deep inside me there was still a lack of joy.

Then I found Christ, and learned about God's love for me and his incredible grace. I discovered God's wisdom in his word and read amazing scriptures. My life changed drastically on many levels. I thought differently about things, and my circle of friends also changed. The things that were important to me in the past were not that important anymore. It's not that my life was suddenly easier or simpler, but it had more meaning. I felt I had direction and that I belonged somewhere. I knew that God wanted me to be happy. He said so in his word: "Delight yourself in the Lord and he will give you the desires of your heart" (Psalm 37:4 NIV).

What were the desires of my heart? I wanted a great husband. I wanted a good job. I wanted good, healthy children. I wanted friends who knew and understood me. I wanted to earn enough money, not a lot, just enough. I wanted the right house in the right neighbourhood. These were the desires of my heart, and once I had these I knew my life would be complete and that I would feel fulfilled. Well, God was very good to me. I can honestly say that every dream I had was fulfilled. I married a wonderful man, and had two beautiful and healthy children. I got a great teaching job at a good school, and we lived comfortably in a nice house situated in a good neighbourhood. We made friends with some wonderfully sincere people in our congregation, who had only our best interests at heart. God truly blessed us in so many ways.

Becoming a wife and a mother was wonderful, but also very tough at times. Juggling a household, motherhood, and a job was very challenging and often I would lose sight of what life was all about. I often had to stop and remind myself of all the great things that God had done in my life, and how grateful I should be. I had no reason to feel discontented with my life, and yet, I am ashamed to say, something was lacking. I felt guilty about it and wouldn't share these feelings with anyone. When Dave suggested that we should maybe move away from the "rat race" to a smaller town, where we could experience more quality of life, I was very keen. Maybe this was where I would find true joy.

God opened all the doors for us, and within a month we had moved to a beautiful coastal town on the "Garden Route", the most beautiful stretch of coastline in South Africa. Almost immediately, both Dave and I found jobs and the kids settled into their new environment very well. Life was perfect. We spent beautiful days on the beach and watched many colourful sunsets. We joined a great church and made some new friends. We had so many new dreams and ambitions ... It's funny how quickly life can get busy – household, motherhood, and work. Why was I still lacking that inner peace and joy? What was wrong with me?

Almost exactly a year later, the symptoms of my illness started, and by the end of that year the diagnosis of MND was made. And that's when it happened: at this very tragic and uncertain time of my life, God gave me the peace I had so long longed for. I was sad and shocked, but for the first time I felt a peace in my heart that I had not experienced before. This peace brought me joy, not the "ha ha" kind of happy joy, but a deep inner joy in knowing that God was there, knowing that this illness was not my battle to fight but God's plan with a purpose. The Creator of the universe had a plan and purpose with *me.* I know it sounds strange, but this made me feel so special and loved.

It has now been four years of deterioration and weakening, of tears and frustration at times. But also a time of growing in faith, purpose, love, grace, understanding, and joy; a deepening in old relationships and the beginning of new ones; experiencing the freedom that comes from having hope, of not having to be pulled down by the burdens of life.

> *I have told you these things, so that in me you may have peace. In this world you will have trouble. But take heart! I have overcome the world.*

JOHN 16:33 NIV

May the God of hope fill you with all joy and peace as you trust in him, so that you may overflow with hope by the power of the Holy Spirit.

ROMANS 15:13 NIV

I can't help but go back to the scripture that I first quoted, from Psalm 37: "Delight yourself in the Lord and he will give you the desires of your heart." What does that mean? I think often we confuse the desires of the heart with the desires of the flesh. Why do I want a good husband? So that I will feel loved and secure. Why do I want good, obedient children? So I will be seen as a good parent, and that will make me feel confident and secure. Why do I want the perfect job and salary? So I will not lack anything and feel secure, and so that I can make friends with the right kind of people. Why do I want to live in the right neighbourhood and have the right kind of friends? So that I will feel loved and enjoy a sense of belonging. Why do I desire all these things? So I can be happy and live a meaningful life.

Is it wrong for me to want this? No. However, it is wrong to place your joy and hope in all of these things, because you will always be disappointed and feel unfulfilled. We are trained from childhood to rely on people, things, and circumstances to make us happy. We were created for one purpose only, and that is to bring glory to God. Only when we fulfil that purpose, regardless of our circumstances, will we find true peace and joy. Only God loves us with a perfect love. He is our Protector, our Comforter, and our Refuge. We can only delight in him.

Recently, a friend of mine, who went through a painful divorce a number of years ago, commented that she didn't know how to find joy in her life again. There are so many others just like her, experiencing life's challenges and trials. There is an answer though: only God can give you joy. Ask him. "Restore to me the joy of your salvation and grant me a willing spirit, to sustain me" (Psalm 51:12 NIV).

> *Though the fig tree does not bud and there are no grapes on the vines, though the olive crop fails and the fields produce no food, though there are no sheep in the pen and no cattle in the stalls, yet I will rejoice in the Lord, I will be joyful in God my Saviour.*
>
> HABAKKUK 3:17–18 NIV

> *Though you have not seen him, you love him; and even though you do not see him now, you believe in him and are filled with an inexpressible and glorious joy, for you are receiving the goal of your faith, the salvation of your souls.*
>
> 1 PETER 1:8–9 NIV

CHAPTER 19

To him who overcomes

The love of many will grow cold. But the one who endures to the end will be saved.

JESUS CHRIST

Jozanne's Story

Recently a friend of mine emailed me in response to my previous email "Give me Joy":

> *"Restore to me the joy of your salvation and grant me a willing spirit, to sustain me..." (Psalm 51:12 NIV). Thank you for this scripture. I can relate to everything you mentioned, apart from finding the peace and the joy, as my life is a roller coaster of emotions as I seek joy from the flesh. I am finding myself distant from God, and people in general. I pray that I will find God as you have, and pray for us as a family to find God. It is not God who has moved. We have ...*

I know what it feels like to be far from God. I have been there many times. The worst part is that it makes you feel so guilty ... and guilt doesn't really help to make you feel closer to God. As you know, God is as close to you now as he was the day you were saved. His love and passion for you have not changed one bit. The only thing that has changed is your *perception* of how he feels about you. Our minds are our worst enemy: that is where Satan has the most power over us. That's why God says: "Be transformed by the renewing of your mind" (Romans 12:2 NIV).

I know that you know this. I always did too, but what does it mean and how do we live it? I have only learned this now. Something about my illness makes me feel very loved by God, and this feeling of love seems to override all other feelings I used to have in the past, such as guilt, fear, and uncertainty. It's not only an *understanding* of God's love for me because of what Jesus did so many years ago ... It is a knowing of God's love for me because of what he does in my life *now!*

You might wonder what he could possibly be doing in my life, seeing that I am basically paralysed and have a terminal illness, but, you see, that's where the beauty lies. Because I am completely helpless, I *know* that without God I would not be able to live for one day. (None of us can. But we don't live like this, we all rely so much on ourselves and think that God is only there for the stuff we can't deal with. We live as though we don't need him for EVERYTHING.)

He is the reason I can cope with my life, and not only cope but have joy and peace. I see his hand in everything, which makes me continually grateful. But you don't have to be ill to see God's hand in your life; it's just an advantage I have. When I was still healthy, I often gave myself the credit for things because I could do the small stuff. I only consulted God for the big things, and when I couldn't cope with the small stuff I would try harder, get tired, fail, and feel guilty. In the end, I would be so focused on everything I was or wasn't doing that I would lose sight of what God was doing in my life at the time. How can you be grateful for something that you don't see?

My mind would tell me that I was disappointing God, which led to guilt and feeling far from God ... Satan then tells you you have to work hard to earn God's love for you again, when in fact, his feelings never changed. We all understand this – but do we *really believe* this? No, we tend to believe the lie. When I read *Revelation,* Jesus repeats many times "to him who overcomes", followed by a number of glorious promises. He doesn't say, "to him who does all things right, and deserves all these promises".

What must we overcome? I have come to believe that it is our minds and perceptions that we have to overcome. We cannot think like the world anymore. For example, to the world, Jesus suffering on the cross makes no sense. In the same way, personal suffering also doesn't make sense.

> *In this you greatly rejoice, though now for a little while you may have had to suffer grief in all kinds of trials. These have come so that your faith – of greater worth than gold, which perishes even though refined by fire – may be proved*

genuine and may result in praise, glory and honour when Jesus Christ is revealed.

1 PETER 1:6–7 NIV

Jesus has already overcome the world; he has won the battle for us already. All we have to do is to overcome Satan's lies, of which the biggest one is: how God feels about us. If only we could realize that nothing we have ever done, or will do, will in any way earn for us what Christ has done for us. If we understand that, then even our worst day spiritually will not lead to feelings of guilt, but rather a feeling of gratitude for God's great and unconditional love for us, despite our sin. Gratitude is the only feeling that can truly motivate and sustain our relationship with God.

For Christ's love compels us, because we are convinced that one died for all, and therefore all died. And he died for all, that those who live should no longer live for themselves but for him who died for them and was raised again.

2 CORINTHIANS 5:14–15 NIV

My illness helps me daily to be grateful. I am grateful for the people in my life, for the care and love we receive, for all our needs that are met as a family. I am grateful for the time that I can spend with Dave and the kids as, together, we prepare for the day that I won't be around anymore. I am grateful for the special conversations I can have with my family and all those I love. I am grateful for so many things, but more than anything, I am grateful for the grace I receive that leads to the hope I have, and that brings the calming peace that I experience. All this makes me feel close to God, and I am so thankful for that.

> *Therefore, I urge you, brothers, in view of God's mercy, to offer your bodies as living sacrifices, holy and pleasing to God – this is your spiritual act of worship. Do not conform any longer to the pattern of this world, but be transformed by the renewing of your mind. Then you will be able to test and approve what God's will is – his good, pleasing and perfect will.*
>
> ROMANS 12:1–2 NIV

So when and why do we feel far from God? I know for me it's when I lose sight of the bigger picture, and start believing lies like: "You need more to be happy"; "Life should be easier than this"; "God doesn't hear my prayers"; "I have messed up too much". The lies are subtle and seem so true, especially when we look at facts or when we compare ourselves to others, but that is when we need to overcome by renewing our minds. This is where we need to hold on to what is true – not man's truth, but God's truth.

Remember that this life is not our final destination. Remember that we live in a broken world, and that all that is bad will pass, but so too will all that is good. Don't get too attached to this world because it will not last, but rather live your life every day, one day at a time, in gratitude and in truth.

> *To him who overcomes, I will give the right to sit with me on my throne, just as I overcame and sat with my Father on his throne.*

REVELATION 3:21 NIV

CHAPTER 20

Is there a shortcut?

It is our great illusion that life is a property to be owned or an object to be grasped, that people can be managed or manipulated.

HENRI NOUWEN[31]

The real question is, "Do I live my losses for my sake or for Jesus' sake?" The choice is a choice for death or for life...

HENRI NOUWEN[32]

"Live your life every day, one day at a time, in gratitude and truth," Jozanne writes, and in her last chapter she will write about completing her Everest climb. There's no pretending it is going to be easy, but we are convinced that it will be worth it – because we have the promises of Revelation "to him who overcomes". However, we live in a world where many

---

31 Henri Nouwen, Turn my mourning into dancing, © 2001, Thomas Nelson, Nashville.

32 Henri Nouwen, Our Second Birth, © 1998, 2006, Crossroad Publishing Co., New York.

are seeking a shortcut to the end. At the time of writing, the British media is awash with items to do with assisted suicide. There have been two court cases with conflicting outcomes, and there has been a passionate advocacy for "assisted death", as he calls it, by the novelist Terry Pratchett, in the 2010 Richard Dimbleby lecture. He has the right to speak as he suffers from a rare form of Alzheimer's disease, from which, if allowed to run its course, he will eventually die. His sound-bite summary was, "My life, my death, my choice." It would be fair to say that it represents the view of many, probably the majority, of the British public. It's the individual's right, especially in the face of a degenerating terminal illness, to choose when they have had enough, when to die.

However, is that the case? What are we to think? There are two "C"s which most frequently appear in the argument for making assisted suicide legal, and they sound very persuasive. They are "Compassion" and "Choice". Together, they are a potent combination. After all, who could reasonably stand against them? Aren't Christians meant to be compassionate? And aren't we called to be free?

A friend said to me, "The Bible's not all that helpful. The two examples of suicide (Ahithophel and Judas) pass without comment..." That's true, but that doesn't mean that the Bible has nothing to say about it. It is anyway dangerous to generalize from particular examples (of which there are probably seven, none of which has a neat moral verdict attached). We do better by looking at principles within the Bible story. Genesis 1 and 2 lay down the foundational principle: "then the Lord God formed the man of dust from the ground and breathed into his nostrils the breath of life, and the man became a living creature." (2:7) In other words, life was God's gift to man, and cherishing the creation was his mandate (1:28). In Genesis 4, the story of Cain and Abel, the consequences of taking life are twice spelled out (verses 11 and 12, and 15). The principle is made explicit: "You shall not murder"[33] in the Ten Commandments (Exodus 20:13). Life is God's gift; it is not for humans to take it away. When Job hears of his children's death, his response is: "Naked I came from my mother's womb, and naked shall I return. The Lord gave, and the Lord has taken away; blessed be the name of the Lord." (Job 1:21) It's as if he says, "Well, the giving of life is the Lord's prerogative, and so is its taking. That's his business." These are archetypal stories, establishing the backdrop for understanding subsequent scriptures.

Nevertheless, didn't Jesus introduce a new and less severe code? One thing is certain, and that is he did not do away with the Ten Commandments:

> *For truly, I say to you, until heaven and earth pass away, not an iota, not a dot, will pass from the Law until all is accomplished. Therefore, whoever relaxes one of the least of these com-*

---

33 The Hebrew word includes causing death through carelessness or negligence.

> *mandments and teaches others to do the same will be called least in the kingdom of heaven, but whoever does them and teaches them will be called great in the kingdom of heaven.*
>
> MATTHEW 5:18–19

If anything, he strengthens the prohibition on murder, all within the Sermon on the Mount. Nowhere do we find him approving of the taking of life. It's inconceivable. It is true that he treats sinners with love and forgiveness (e.g. John 8), but he does not excuse the sin or abrogate the command. We might fairly conclude that he would not be in the queue to condemn the depressive driven to take their own life, but he might well condemn the society which fails to care for them. He says his mission is to bring life, "life in all its fullness" (John 10:10).[34] St Paul tells the Christians in Corinth not to abuse their bodies, because the Holy Spirit is in them. "You are not your own" (1 Corinthians 6:19).

The most important consideration of all, however, is the fact that "The Word became flesh and dwelt among us" (John 1:14). Humans were created "in the image of God", and God himself actually became a human being. This confers an infinite value, a sanctity, on every life. It's not that everyone is divine, or part of God, but everyone is precious; everyone has digni-

---

34 New Century Version, © 2005 Thomas Nelson, Inc.

ty. So in the parable of the sheep and goats, the king, who clearly is Jesus, says to the sheep, "Truly, I say to you, as you did it to one of the least of these my brothers, you did it to me" (Matthew 25:40). Every living person (not least the weakest and most marginalized) deserves the respect we would afford to Jesus himself. The implication for a Christian couldn't be clearer.

However, not everyone is a Christian. We live in a mixed society. Opinion formers in education and the media, lawmakers in government, and the multitudes on social networking sites do not share the same presuppositions. Have we anything to say to which they would be able to relate, other than what Terry Pratchett called "the God bit"? We should not be ashamed of the God bit. But I'm sure we have more to say, though it has to be expressed in a Christ-like manner; in other words, not with harsh self-righteousness or condemnation. There is no doubt that those who are facing the issues of terminal illness, or crippling disability, or chronic pain are up against a fearful mountain, and that those who speak for them are passionate in their concern to ease their lot.

So what about the two Cs – Compassion and Choice – which are often cited as reasons for assisted suicide? Compassion concerns the people who surround the "sufferer"; family, carers, friends, and onlookers. Choice is more about the individual who is affected.

CHAPTER 21

Compassion costs

Let us not underestimate how hard it is to be compassionate. Compassion is hard because it requires the inner disposition to go with others to the place where they are weak, vulnerable, lonely, and broken. But this is not our spontaneous response to suffering. What we desire most is to do away with suffering by fleeing from it or finding a quick cure for it.

HENRI NOUWEN[35]

Compassion, it is argued, dictates that we should put people out of their misery. "I wouldn't let my dog suffer like this." In the UK this view seemed to be backed up by the Crown Prosecution Service when it included being "wholly motivated by compassion" as a mitigating factor in assisting in someone's death. But compassion is not the same as pity; it's more than feeling sorry for someone. "I can't bear watching this any longer" can easily be mistaken for compassion; in other words, it's more to do with the onlook-

35 Henri Nouwen, The Way of the Heart, © 1981 Harper Collins, New York.

ers' feelings for themselves than with their feeling for the other person. Its original meaning is "suffering with", which is a much stronger quality. That's more like standing alongside, sticking with the sufferer to the end. With the discovery that we can have some form of communication with some patients in a persistent vegetative state (deep and long-lasting unconsciousness), one of the first questions journalists asked was whether that meant one could get an answer to the question, "Do you want to go on living?" They expected, I think, to be told "No", and that this would solve the dilemma of keeping comatose patients expensively alive, but the surprising truth they heard was that the vast majority of "locked-in" patients (perhaps the nearest one can get to a conscious vegetative state) want to stay alive.* Contrary to the account in the film, Jean-Dominique Bauby, who authored *The Diving Bell and the Butterfly* merely by a movement of an eyelid, did not ask for his life to be ended.[36] Just down the road from where we once lived, in Stepping Hill Hospital, is a twenty-six-year-old mother locked in her body, Michelle Wheatley, who steadfastly wants to live. There is, it seems, a deep-seated instinct to stay alive, and actually to keep alive. We don't naturally stand and do nothing when someone tries to jump under a train. Something tells us that life is precious. We know it's good to be alive, even when it's hard. We value life, rightly.

---

36 The Independent, 6 February 2010.

[* Source: http://www.alis-asso.fr/e_upload/pdf/quality_of_life_in_locked_in_syndrome_survivors_a.bruno_f.pellas_s._laureys.pdf]

We live in a culture of fear, which is profoundly unhealthy. We are a society dogged by fear: fear of terrorism, pandemic, financial and environmental catastrophe, and personal insecurity. The campaign for assisted suicide feeds on and fuels fear. The fear it feeds on is our innate fear of pain and dying. These are situations of loss of control. Suicide gives an illusion of ultimate control. "This at least I can decide and do." The irony of course is that it is in fact the ultimate surrender of control. There is no more control possible. There are, however, more human ways of facing the fear. It is possible to assert value, dignity, creativity, and life. Beethoven, in his deafness, and Van Gogh, in his depression, defied their disabilities. In September 1888 Van Gogh wrote to his sister Willemien, "...we need good cheer and happiness, hope and love. The uglier, older, meaner, iller, poorer I get, the more I wish to take my revenge by doing brilliant colour, well arranged, resplendent."* Fear of suffering saps the will to live. Strangely, suffering can have the opposite effect, as Jozanne soberly and amply demonstrates.

[* Ed. Leo Jansen, Hans Luijten, and Nienke Bakker, Vincent Van Gogh: The Complete Letters; Thames and Hudson, London, 2009. Retrieved from http://vangoghletters.org/vg/]

Don't mistake me. Pain, suffering, and dying are terrible, but letting them rule our actions and laws is even more so. A country that does that has lost its way. The answer is not to surrender life, but to fight against pain, as doctors have long dedicated themselves to doing, and to have the compassion to "ease" death's coming. Exactly what that means is the substance of the debate about the end of life, for a further fear the campaign fuels is for the old and ill, who feel themselves becoming "a burden" to their families, or even to the state. "Maybe I ought to end it and relieve them..." There is a danger of self-imposed pressure, or subtle external expectation being applied to the vulnerable, if assisted suicide becomes a legal option. Indeed, in the wake of Terry Pratchett's lecture in the UK, this was explicitly enunciated by figures as articulate as Baroness Warnock and A.N. Wilson. "Yes, the elderly are a burden; of course they are." They are no longer economically productive; they cost the rest of society money; they cause their family anxiety and pain. "Burden" is not a neutral word. A burden is a nuisance, something you want to get rid of – the archetype in literature, I suppose, is Christian in *Pilgrim's Progress,* who was mightily relieved when his burden rolled away. In the context of people, the message is chilling. They are a burden, whom we would be better off without. This is a world away from honouring the past contribution and present wisdom of the elderly, or loving the vulnerable.

The financial issue is admittedly a real one. It may seem as if health care is a sacred cow in politics, with every UK party promising to ring-fence it, but with ever-increasing costs in treatments, and an aging population, I have no doubt that there will eventually be effective cuts in the health budget, with the financial crisis having so massively increased national debts. A simple cost-cutting measure would be to legalize euthanasia. Indeed, Ludwig Minelli of the Dignitas "clinic" in Switzerland gave economics as one of the reasons for assisting suicide. It would save the NHS money clearing up after failed attempts, let alone the costs of long-term care. Doctors certainly need to beware of officiously keeping alive, and somehow society needs to confirm that. But the reason for assisted suicide saving money is a betrayal of values, betrayal in both its meanings: it would betray what our values really are, cash above life; and it would betray our human values, which hold life as the most precious gift there is.

The relationship between doctor and patient lies at the heart of good medical practice. It needs to be a relationship of trust. If the role of life-ender is added to that of life-enhancer and life-preserver in the doctor's remit, that fundamentally changes the relationship. "This person, who is caring for me today, yesterday terminated another patient's life and they might try to persuade me..." Once assisted death is added to the list of possible available "treatments", we have redefined the role of doctor, and opened the door to a brave but sinister new world. It is naïve to equate symptom or pain relief which may shorten life, with the intention to end life. There is a categorical distinction between the two, the difference of intention. There is a world apart: the doctor becomes a dealer in death, a grim reaper, rather than a guardian of life. Palliative care, relieving discomfort, pain and fear in the terminally and chronically ill, is the final gift of medicine to the patient. It's well, though not fully nor equally, developed in Britain. A political platform worth fighting for would be to expand and resource it fully. It's admittedly a costly option, because now the state gets it on the cheap as it is largely charitably funded.

We need to assert the intrinsic value of life. The campaign for assisted suicide talks a lot about quality of life, and plays on the assumption that fit, healthy, "normal" lives are of a higher quality than those, for example, of the disabled or terminally ill. In one sense, it's right. The disabled and dying would no doubt choose to be "normal" (of course, I would rather be fit and live longer; Jozanne would love to see her children grow up!); but for the most part, they would by no means regard their lives as without value. Far less should the rest of society so treat them. Even the utterly dependent disabled child has value, as the child of her parents, and as the recipient of love and self-sacrificing care. That might be her only contribution to society, but that is the greatest contribution there is, being the indicator of that society's compassion and humanity.

As previous chapters in this book have shown, dependence on others is not the unmitigated ill it's sometimes painted. Of course, all human life, all life itself, is interdependent, and to put it bluntly having your nappy changed at sixty years old is no more undignified than at six months. After all, we all depend on others to clean up our mess after us, one way or another. Behold, the lowly dung beetle!

CHAPTER 22

My life ... my choice

...for why, said he [Giant Despair], should you choose life, seeing it is attended with so much bitterness?

JOHN BUNYAN[37]

In *My Donkeybody* I devoted some pages (in Chapter 22, Enigma) to addressing one issue, that is, the personal cost to those involved in the act of assisted suicide, whether carers, family, or health professionals. Since then I have met Debbie Purdy who has Multiple Sclerosis and has fought through the British (and European) courts in order, basically, to ensure her husband, Omar, would not have to face prosecution if he took her to a facility where she could take her own life. Eventually, in July 2009, she won a ruling that guidelines concerning prosecution for assisted suicide should be published. We spent a large part of a day discussing the issues. We are in very similar boats, but we have quite different views. The BBC was interested to see if we could come up with a "compromise" proposal. Well, it wasn't long enough!

---

37 Pilgrim's Progress, James Nisbet, London, 1880.

But we were able to realize that we were very much human beings, for whom what we shared far outweighed our differences. One lesson I learned that day was not to create a monster out of an "opponent". We left as friends.

A central theme of those who argue for "assisted dying" is their right to choose. How can anyone object? It's my life, the argument runs; so who has the right to curtail, control, what I choose to do with it, including when I choose to end it? Autonomy, or the right to determine one's own life and destiny, is often regarded as an unquestioned and inalienable good. Yet along with every right goes responsibility.

> *No man is an island, entire of itself; every man is a piece of the continent, a part of the main. If a clod be washed away by the sea, Europe is the less, as well as if a promontory were, as well as if a manor of thy friend's or of thine own were: any man's death diminishes me, because I am involved in mankind, and therefore never send to know for whom the bells tolls; it tolls for thee.*[38]

John Donne's well-known statement of human interdependence might well read, "Thy death diminishes every man." Our choices affect others. For instance, the choice to take one's own life affects one's family and friends, whether it's in helping with the act or in dealing with the feelings of loss and guilt afterwards

38 Meditation 17

("If only I'd shown I cared more..."). It also affects the medical and caring professions, whose raison d'être is to preserve life. To demand they compromise their vocation for one's own purposes is too high a cost. In addition, it affects others who are vulnerable, as it puts physician-assisted death on the menu of possible "treatments" for disability, degenerative illness, and even extreme old age. Society is more than a collection of individuals; it's a community of people, each of whom matters. There is something fundamentally selfish in insisting on one's own rights and wishes at the expense of others.

We see the same argument in another context in the woman's "right to choose" whether to have a termination of her unborn child. An opposition is proposed between the Pro-Choice movement and the Pro-Life movement. You are either pro-choice or pro-life (of which, the sub-text is, you are in favour of freedom or in favour of legalism). In fact, as the beginning of this book and its title suggest, you can be both! You can, like Thérèse Martin, "choose everything", that is, embrace *all* that life brings. In choosing the singing of the group "Musica Secreta" as her inheritance track on Radio 4's *Saturday Live* programme, novelist Sarah Dunant sketched the background of the hidden music in the courts and convents of renaissance Italy, and said as they sang, "these women singing now are tasting joy and triumph as much as they are trying to rebel against incarceration; and I think that's what people do in all difficult situations in their life. Times get tough but they find a way to find just some joy in it to keep them going ... Not everything that happens in life is wonderful. Along with the glamour and the pleasure, there are some very tough things. But even the tough things in life – you can find some joy in them. You don't need to be defeated by them."[39] Degenerative illness and disability are a real incarceration, but there is more joy to be found within it, than anticipating its end.

Terry Pratchett said, "If I knew that I could die at any time I wanted, then suddenly every day would be as precious as a million pounds." I found this logic hard to follow: for me every day is infinitely precious, especially since my diagnosis. Every morning I wake up to a mixture of challenges and surprises, to another day of life. Alison Davis has spina bifida, hydrocephalus, emphysema, osteoporosis, and arthritis. She desperately wanted a child, and had to come to terms with the knowledge that she never would.

> *I have severe pain every day, and ... morphine doesn't always alleviate it. I also have crushed and fractured vertebra, caused by my osteoporotic bones, which means additional pain ... Twenty-five years ago, I ... decided I wanted to die, a settled and entirely competent death wish that lasted for 10 years. During those years I attempted suicide more than once. On the occasion I best remember, I was treated against my will by doc-*

---

39 BBC Radio 4, Saturday Live, 6 February 2010.

> *tors, who saved my life. Then, I was very angry with the doctors who saved my life, but now I'm extremely grateful. Yet because of the requirements of the Mental Capacity Act, and the Director of Public Prosecutions' new guidelines, if similar circumstances obtained now, I would be left to die...*
>
> *But I would actually have missed the best years of my life, notwithstanding pain that is worse now than it was when I wanted to die. No one would ever have known that the future held something better for me, not in terms of physical ability, but in terms of support and the love of friends who refused to accept my view that my life was "over".*
>
> *It's very easy to give up on a body as "broken" as ... mine, and it can be tough to continue. But it is possible to come out the other side of a death wish, to use well the time that would otherwise have been lost, and to demonstrate that life is precious and worth living, despite many serious challenges.*[40]

If one could sum up this attitude, which has no illusions about our choosing to be born, and doesn't demand to control the time of our dying, it might be: "My life, my death, my adventure." One of the two mottoes for the State of South Carolina is "*Dum spiro,*

---

40 Letter to The Independent newspaper, 1 February 2010, quoted by kind permission of the author.

spero" ("While I breathe, I hope", or more familiarly, "Where there's life, there's hope"). It's thought to date back to Roman times. In our day, we are in danger of replacing it with *"Dum spiro, timeo"* as the motto for our society: "While I breathe, I'm afraid." We are increasingly ruled by fear. We are frightened of the unexpected, of the unknown, of what we can't control. We are stressed-out, risk-averse control freaks! How deeply and inhumanly sad! How different from God who repeatedly in the Bible says, "Fear not!" And that, I suppose, is the crux of the matter. Where faith has drained away, fear seeps in to take its place. Faith says, "Even though I walk through the valley of the shadow of death, I will fear no evil, for you are with me" (Psalm 23:4).

On 4 October 2009 Rowan Williams, the Archbishop of Canterbury, preached a harvest sermon in a small country church in Blean in Kent. He talked about St Francis, who is commemorated that day.

> *He saw the universe around him as a set of relationships in which he had a share. The objects he encountered each day were part of a great complex circle of life in which he as a human being had a vital and unique role – but not the role of sole manager and proprietor.*
>
> *In other words, he wasn't afraid of not being in charge. And that fearlessness is expressed in so many aspects of his life – in the risks he took in reaching out to outcasts and people with dangerous diseases, in his insistence on living simply*

and relying only on other people's charity, even in his courageous acceptance of pain and death – "Sister Death", not a terrifying thing that denied human dignity but just another feature of this astonishing and uncontrollable world. He had learned the great lesson of Jesus Christ himself, that the biggest difference is made by those who are strong enough and secure enough to let go and to forget the dreams of total power.

Three months later, on the first anniversary of my retirement, a friend with Multiple Sclerosis whose husband with MND had died a year previously wrote to me from Australia: "I realised a long time ago that no matter how we push and pull at ourselves in regard to our life path, at the end of the day we just have to hold God's hand and let HIM help us through it...! I know it is sometimes easier said than done." She is right, and this is living life to the full.

CHAPTER 23

The climb

You have chosen the roughest road, but it leads straight to the hilltops.

JOHN BUCHAN[41]

Jozanne's Story

In the Bible, the Christian walk or journey is referred to as running a race. Paul said, "However, I consider my life worth nothing to me, if only I may *finish the race* and complete the task the Lord Jesus has given me – the task of testifying to the gospel of God's grace" (Acts 20:24 NIV).

When I read this, I don't think of a 100 metre sprint but rather a long-distance marathon. I think of the Comrades' Marathon that is run in South Africa every year. Thousands of people take part from all over the world, but there can only be one winner or one person who gets to finish first. So obviously, people don't all run to come first. The victory lies in completing this challenging race. Many do finish the race, but every year there are many who don't. There

---

41 Greenmantle, Chapter 1.

are thousands more though, who, every year, watch the Comrades and then set themselves the goal to run the following year – but never do. This is what the Christian life is like. Many run, but many don't finish; and yet more claim that one day they will run, but then they never do.

I live in George, a town at the foot of the Outeniqua Mountains. From my garden I have a great view of one of the peaks of the mountain. Some days it looks bright and clear, and you can almost see every rock, bush, and crevice. On other days, it looks blue and hazy, and sometimes it is covered in a blanket of clouds. It's so easy to go for days without even noticing the mountain. You get caught up in being busy and all you notice are the houses, buildings, and traffic lights around you, but it takes only a ten-minute drive, out of town, to see what is so obvious, that the mountain is so big and the town so small. It puts things back into perspective for me, and provides me with a sense of peace, knowing that there is more to life than just me and my problems. Life is bigger than that. The mountain is bigger than that.

I admire mountain climbers. People don't climb mountains because it's easy, but because it's rewarding. The victory lies in completing the climb, in reaching the top. I know what that feels like. In 1997, Dave and I were living in Cape Town. I was about four months pregnant with Luke when a group of us decided to climb Table Mountain, or let me rather say, walk up Table Mountain. Most people, especially tourists, make use of the cable car system to ascend the mountain while taking in the spectacular views of the city, ocean, and harbour – a trip we had made and enjoyed together at least twice before. This time, however, we looked forward to the challenge of climbing and walking up. Although I was pregnant, I was healthy, and there was no risk involved. The pregnancy just added to the challenge for me, and increased my desire to be victorious and to reach the top. The hike only took about two hours, and along the way I was huffing and puffing like an old steam train, but I made it. I reached the top. It was wonderful.

This, I know, is nothing compared to climbing a mountain like Mount Everest. Real mountain climbers have to prepare months and even years in advance. They have to be fully equipped for any situation that may come their way. They have to carry all their food and water with them, and make sure that their nutritional needs are met to ensure that they have the energy required to complete the gruelling task. They often have to face great obstacles like rock falls or an avalanche; therefore, they have to be focused, determined, and brave, and willing to make any sacrifice necessary to compete the climb, even risking their lives. To the normal man on the street this might not make sense but, to the climbing community, the great rewards in climbing a mountain are so clear and obvious.

For me, another way of looking at the Christian journey is like climbing a mountain. It is definitely not easy, but the reward at the end of journey is so incredible. Each of us will have our own mountain to climb. Some of us will have Mount Everest to climb, while others may only have to walk up Table Mountain. It doesn't matter how big or small the mountain, the reward far outweighs any effort or sacrifice made, and the victory lies in overcoming the obstacles and reaching the summit. "Whatever you do, work at it with all your heart, as working for the Lord, not for men, since you know that you will receive an inheritance from the Lord as a reward. It is the Lord Christ you are serving" (Colossians 3:23–24 NIV).

Just like a climber, to complete the Christian journey, we need to be well prepared and equipped. God has graciously given us everything we need to be victorious. "All Scripture is God-breathed and is useful for teaching, rebuking, correcting and training in righteousness, so that the man of God may be *thoroughly equipped* for every good work" (2 Timothy 3:16–17 NIV).

For the journey, we need to be well nourished. "Then Jesus declared, 'I am the *bread of life.* He who comes to me will never go hungry, and he who believes in me will never be thirsty'" (John 6:35 NIV).

We must be focused, determined, and brave.

> *Therefore, since we are surrounded by such a great cloud of witnesses, let us throw off everything that hinders and the sin that so easily entangles, and let us* run with perseverance *the race marked out for us. Let us* fix our eyes *on Jesus, the author and perfecter of our faith, who for the joy set before him endured the cross, scorning its shame, and sat down at the right hand of the throne of God. Consider him who endured such opposition from sinful men, so that you will not grow weary and lose heart.*
>
> HEBREWS 12:1–3 NIV

I have been climbing my mountain for about fifteen years now. Most of those years were spent in the base camp, at the foot of my mountain, where I know God was preparing me. I was always afraid to climb and thought the base camp was my goal. I didn't think I could make it to the top, but God showed me, through my illness, that it wasn't about me, or what I could do. It has always been about him. "It is God who arms me with strength and makes my way perfect. He makes my feet like the feet of a deer; *he enables me* to stand on the heights" (2 Samuel 22:33–34 NIV).

I finally left the base camp and started my ascent. God has chosen Mount Everest for me. It definitely has not been easy, and my foot has often slipped. I have often felt weary and at times I didn't think I could go any further. Parts of this climb are very steep and far beyond anything I could achieve, but he continues to show me his power and strength, and when I'm tired, he is there. "...but those who hope in the LORD will renew their strength. They will soar on wings like eagles; they will run and not grow weary, they will walk and not be faint" (Isaiah 40:31 NIV).

My climb is nearly over. I think I am near the summit of my mountain. The higher climbers go, the closer they get to the summit, and the harder it becomes to breathe. The oxygen level decreases as the altitude increases, which causes climbers to suffer from altitude sickness. (According to the Internet, *Symptoms of mild and moderate altitude sickness typically consist of headache, shortness of breath, sleeping trouble, loss of appetite, nausea, and rapid pulse.)* As the muscles of the body weaken with the progression of Motor Neurone Disease, so too do the muscles necessary for breathing become weaker. I feel short of breath, have regular headaches, have trouble sleeping, and often experience a very rapid pulse. But it doesn't worry me, because I know I am nearly at the top of my mountain. The climb is becoming tough now, but I must push on. The reward that awaits me when I complete the climb, far outweighs any sacrifice one makes. Ask any mountain climber!

So here I stand, looking up. The end is in sight and my heart races with excitement. I look forward to the day when I can say: "I have fought the good fight, I have finished the race, I have kept the faith" (2 Timothy 4:7 NIV).

CHAPTER 24

Henceforth

Death be not proud, though some have callèd thee
Mighty and dreadful, for thou art not so...
One short sleep past, we wake eternally,
And death shall be no more; death, thou shalt die.

JOHN DONNE[42]

A well-known brand of cream cheese ran a whole series of commercials with actresses dressed in sheets and wings. Against a backdrop of white fluffy clouds and a blue sky a blonde "angel" sits down saying, "Another perfect day. If only there was something a little different to brighten it up..." Suddenly, there appears a tub of a rather unappetizing new combination of the cheese, and she says, "Now this ... is heaven." The advert ends with the voice-over: "A new spin on a little taste of heaven." Of course, it's a humorous treatment of stereotypical clichés. Yet I suspect it's not so far removed from the vague ideas of heaven held by many in the post-Christian West. It's

---

42 "Holy Sonnet" 10

all perfect, but to be honest, it's all a bit boring. And, frankly, it's rather laughable and unbelievable. Is this really the goal that Jozanne has been heading for – and me? Or, anything remotely like it? If so, it would come nowhere near making the climb worth it. But we are looking forward to something utterly different and utterly wonderful – spending eternity in the company of the One who loved us and gave himself for us.

We both have declared many times, "I believe ... in the resurrection of the dead and life everlasting" (Apostles' Creed). But what do we mean? What are we looking forward to? "We look for the resurrection of the dead, and the life of the world to come" (Nicene Creed). This is how the early church summarized what they found in the New Testament. Why are we so confident? In a nutshell, because of the best attested fact in history: Jesus was raised from the dead. As Bishop Tom Wright has shown in his book, *Surprised by Hope,* the resurrection means much more than merely that we can "go to heaven when we die", though it does mean that. What Peter concluded on the day of Pentecost was, "Let all the house of Israel therefore know for certain that God has made him both Lord and Christ, this Jesus whom you crucified." (Acts 2:36) In other words, in the resurrection God confirmed that the kingdom of heaven has come, and Jesus is its King. It's as if the door has been opened: "When you overcame the sharpness of death, you opened the kingdom of heaven to all believers", in the words of the old Latin hymn.

But what exactly are we looking forward to? Tom Wright helpfully writes: "...all Christian language about the future is like a set of signposts pointing into a mist..."[43] He goes on to say that you don't get photographs on signposts. The sign to Letchworth Garden City, for example, will give you some idea of a town (not a city!) with houses, parks possibly, and of course gardens. If you know a bit of history, you will guess that it was planned as a pleasant integrated environment for people to live in, about a century ago. But until you arrive there in the coach you won't know what it's actually like. However, we are not without signposts to the future.

The first signpost is the risen Jesus himself, and the nature of his resurrection body. It tells us that the dead can be raised to new life, and this new life is different from resuscitation in the way that Jesus' body was like but different from the body that had been buried. It was clearly the same body; it still carried the marks of Roman execution. Like a body of our dimensions, he was visible and recognizable; he could cook and eat; he could be touched – and yet like a body of another dimension, he could appear out of thin air and disappear just as suddenly. So

---

43 Tom Wright, Surprised by Hope, SPCK, London, 2007, page 144.

there was continuity and discontinuity in the resurrection body.

The second signpost is what Jesus said to the thief crucified next to him, "Today you will be with me in Paradise." As the thief recognizes Jesus the King and seems to expect the kingdom some time in the future ("when you come in your kingdom"), Jesus by contrast assures him of Paradise that day. When he dies, he will enjoy the company of the king – "today".

The third signpost is what the disciples are told on the Mount of Olives, after Jesus has ascended: "This Jesus, who was taken up from you into heaven, will come in the same way as you saw him go into heaven" (Acts 1:11). It's easy to focus on the "up ... there" (as if it were directions for space travel, which it clearly isn't), whereas the sign actually points to the fact that Jesus will return finally to establish his kingdom. As I noted earlier, Jesus has inaugurated or begun his kingdom on earth, his resurrection has confirmed it, and the church's task is to proclaim and extend it. The final act of establishing the kingdom is described in Revelation 21 and 22: "Then I saw a new heaven and a new earth, for the first heaven and the first earth had passed away, and the sea was no more. And I saw the holy city, new Jerusalem, coming down out of heaven from God, prepared as a bride adorned for her husband" (21:1–2). Here is the new creation of which Jesus' resurrection is the sign, of which he is the "firstfruits". It's unimaginably beautiful; there's no injustice or sin there; and above all God has his dwelling place there: "its temple is the Lord God the Almighty and the Lamb" (21:22).

The impression we get in the New Testament is of Jesus returning, or descending, to establish his reign in a new heaven and earth, more than of an ethereal spiritual world above the bright blue sky. But reminding ourselves that we just have signposts pointing into the mist, or as St Paul put it, "Now we see through a glass, darkly; but then face to face: now I know in part; but then I shall know even as also I am known" (1 Corinthians 13:12 AV) – what can we know about what awaits us? Something immediately follows: "So now faith, hope, and love abide, these three; but the greatest of these is love" (13:13). Love awaits us – and there lies our security and our destiny – in the heart of love.

In two great passages teaching about life after death, 1 Corinthians 15 and 1 Thessalonians 4, Paul deals with questions about life after death. The Christians at Corinth seem unsure whether there is a real resurrection at all, partly because they can't envisage a resurrection body. Paul tells them that, beyond doubt, Jesus was raised from death – and that this is at the heart of the good news which has changed their lives, that Jesus is the Messiah and King over all, "And if Christ has not been raised, your faith is futile and you are still in your sins. Then those also who have fallen asleep in Christ have perished. If in Christ we have hope in this life only, we are of all people most to be pitied" (1 Corinthians 15:17–19).

It's as if he's saying, "Get real, you lot, if you don't have this, you don't have anything." And he's equally impatient with their chuntering about the exact nature of our resurrected bodies: "You foolish person! What you sow does not come to life unless it dies. And what you sow is not the body that is to be, but a bare kernel, perhaps of wheat or of some other grain. But God gives it a body as he has chosen, and to each kind of seed its own body" (15:36–38). In other words, "You're dealing with the great Creator and Re-Creator here. To create a body continuous with but different from the original isn't a problem. He's doing it every day." And as we have seen, that's just what he did with Jesus, whom Paul later calls the "man of heaven". "Just as we have borne the image of the man of dust, we shall also bear the image of the man of heaven" (15:49). The time will come when the Lord Jesus Christ "will transform our lowly body to be like his glorious body, by the power that enables him even to subject all things to himself" (Philippians 3:21), his resurrection authority.

The Thessalonian church seems concerned about Christians who die before Jesus returns finally to establish his kingdom, whom Paul had described as "those who have fallen asleep in Christ". Paul told the Corinthians that the dead would be raised imperishable, "and we shall be changed" (15:52). In a similar passage in 1 Thessalonians 4, he reassures his readers that "those who are asleep" will not be forgotten or left behind. In fact, they will steal a march on those who are still alive. He spells it out: "For the Lord himself will descend from heaven with a cry of command, with the voice of an archangel, and with the sound of the trumpet of God. And the dead in Christ will rise first. Then we who are alive, who are left, will be caught up together with them in the clouds to meet the Lord in the air, and so we will always be with the Lord" (4:16–17).

What does it mean to be asleep? Clearly, it's a way of talking about the state between our death and Jesus' return. It could mean the oblivion of physical sleep. You go to sleep and the next thing you know – you are awake. It could mean simply passing out of the dimension of time into an existence without time. These seem unlikely, as what "asleep" does not seem to mean is being non-existent, or even being unaware. Why else does Jesus say to the thief, "*Today* you will be with me in Paradise"? Or, to his disciples, "In my Father's house there are many dwelling places [homes]. If it were not so, I would have told you; for I am going away to prepare a place for you" (John 14:2[44])? After all, Paul himself is torn between his caring for the churches and his desire "to depart and be with Christ, for that is far better" (Philippians 1:23).

"Asleep" seems to me to mean that our bodies are well and truly dead, but that God has not yet finished with them. When Jesus returns, we will have resurrec-

44 Amplified Version © 1987 The Lockman Foundation.

tion bodies "like his glorious body". This might explain why Jesus says about Jairus' daughter, "The child is not dead, but sleeping", and why he says, "*Talitha cumi*" – "Little girl, I say to you, arise" (Mark 5). He is giving a picture of resurrection, as well as proof of his compassion. Of course, he knows that she is dead, but she is not beyond his reviving touch. The decomposition (or cremation) of bodies is not a problem, whatever Martha reckons! Dust we are and to dust we shall return, but God is the Creator. Our bodies are dead, but in ourselves, we are in a "state of restful happiness", held firmly, as Tom Wright puts it, "within the conscious love of God and the conscious presence of Jesus Christ",[45] while we are waiting for the day of resurrection at our Lord's return.

Jesus prayed this for us: "Father, I desire that they also, whom you have given me, may be with me where I am" (John 17:24). That surely is the Father's desire too. "With me in Paradise", "with Christ, which is far better", "for ever with the Lord": clear in the mists of the future, we have that assurance – and that is more than enough, isn't it!

I want to finish with two quotations. The first is from the vision of heaven by Louise Halling, from which I quoted in *My Donkeybody.* And the second, is Paul's triumphant declaration of the unbreakable power of God's love. Finally, there's an epilogue, "Pity Me Not", by Jozanne.

---

45 ibid, pages 184–85.

Those who struggled on earth to find a true home, at last have a real sense of belonging, a real sense of home, a deep sense of rest – a home where we can eat good food, where there are healing oils and wine and where we are truly satisfied...

We meet people who we saw on our TV screens when they were little children dying from hunger in the sweltering heat.

"Never again will they hunger;
never again will they thirst.
The sun will not beat upon them,
nor any scorching heat.
For the Lamb at the centre of the throne will be their shepherd;
he will lead them to springs of living water.
And God will wipe away every tear from their eyes."
(Revelation 7:15–17)

We are living the real live version of Isaiah's vision: The wolf and the lamb lie down together, and there are streams in the desert!

It is the happiest ending of the most amazing love story ever told, where Jesus, our bridegroom, smiles into our eyes and says to us:

"Arise, my darling,
my beautiful one, and come with me.

See! The winter is past;
the rains are over and gone." (Song of Solomon 2:8–13)

The dream is ended. THIS is the morning!

LOUISE HALLING[46]

That is our hope and expectation.

The Spirit himself bears witness with our spirit that we are children of God, and if children, then heirs – heirs of God and fellow heirs with Christ, provided we suffer with him in order that we may also be glorified with him.

For I consider that the sufferings of this present time are not worth comparing with the glory that is to be revealed to us. For the creation waits with eager longing for the revealing of the sons of God. For the creation was subjected to futility, not willingly, but because of him who subjected it, in hope that the creation itself will be set free from its bondage to corruption and obtain the freedom of the glory of the children of God. For we know that the whole creation has been groaning together in the pains of childbirth until now. And not only the creation, but we ourselves, who have the first fruits of the Spirit, groan inwardly as we wait eagerly for adoption

---

46 Used with the author's permission.

as sons, the redemption of our bodies. For in this hope we were saved. Now hope that is seen is not hope. For who hopes for what he sees? But if we hope for what we do not see, we wait for it with patience.

Likewise the Spirit helps us in our weakness. For we do not know what to pray for as we ought, but the Spirit himself intercedes for us with groanings too deep for words. And he who searches hearts knows what is the mind of the Spirit, because the Spirit intercedes for the saints according to the will of God. And we know that for those who love God all things work together for good, for those who are called according to his purpose. For those whom he foreknew he also predestined to be conformed to the image of his Son, in order that he might be the firstborn among many brothers. And those whom he predestined he also called, and those whom he called he also justified, and those whom he justified he also glorified.

What then shall we say to these things? If God is for us, who can be against us? He who did not spare his own Son but gave him up for us all, how will he not also with him graciously give us all things? Who shall bring any charge against God's elect? It is God who justifies. Who is to condemn? Christ Jesus is the one who died – more than that, who was raised – who is at the right hand of God, who indeed is interceding for us.

Who shall separate us from the love of Christ? Shall tribulation, or distress, or persecution, or famine, or nakedness, or danger, or sword? As it is written,

"For your sake we are being killed all the day long; we are regarded as sheep to be slaughtered."

No, in all these things we are more than conquerors through him who loved us. For I am sure that neither death nor life, nor angels nor rulers, nor things present nor things to come, nor powers, nor height nor depth, nor anything else in all creation, will be able to separate us from the love of God in Christ Jesus our Lord.

ROMAN S 8:16–39, ST PAUL

That is our conviction and our testimony, too.

Epilogue

Pity me not

Pity me not:
For I am the rich one
With treasures stored up in the sky.

Pity me not:
God's Spirit's inside me;
I don't feel alone or afraid.

Pity me not:
Though my body is limp
My spirit soars up there on high.

Pity me not:
Though my life may seem shortened
Today is all we can count on.

Pity me not:
My life may seem useless;
But my Father chose me for His glory.

Pity me not:
My joy is complete,
For my purpose before me is clear.

Pity me not:

For our time in this life
Withers and wastes away.

It's the life after this,
When we stand with the Son
That will last for Eternity

So, pity me not.
No, pity me not:
I'm right where God wants me to be.

JOZANNE MOSS

Appendix

Useful information

At the end of *My Donkeybody* I described in simple terms what Motor Neurone, or Lou Gehrig's, Disease is – or more accurately are, as it's an umbrella term for a number of conditions affecting the motor nerves, which begin in different ways but all end the same. Jozanne has vividly portrayed the experience. I'll not repeat what I wrote then, not least because this book isn't just about ALS/MND; it's about living with any terminal illness and retaining faith. Besides the information is readily accessible on the internet or in the excellent *Motor Neuron Disease: the Facts* by Kevin Talbot and Rachael Marsden.[47]

Support groups

The first thing is to link up with the local support group for your condition. Usually all you need to do is type the disease name with 'association' or 'society' into the search engine, for example: UK – www.mnd association.org; South Africa – www.mnda.org.za; United States – www.alsa.org; Australia – www.mnd aust.asn.au; and the international www.alsmndallian

47 Kevin Talbot, Rachael Marsden, Motor Neuron Disease – the Facts, 2008, Oxford University Press, Oxford

ce.mnda.org.za; United States – www.alsa.org; Australia – www.mndaust.asn.au; and the international www.alsmndalliance.org. In our experience, it is hard to overstate the usefulness of such groups. They often include people of supportive faith, and actually sharing with others who are in similar situations is a two-way blessing both for those with the disease and those caring for them. Their websites have a wealth of well tried is a two-way blessing both for those with the disease and those caring for them. Their websites have a wealth of welltried medical and practical information. The UK association has always been my first port of call.

More general patient websites can be a mixed blessing in my opinion, as they're something of a free-for-all, which means you come across scare stories and quack remedies that undermine rather than increase faith. This is especially true of those that rely on advertising for income. I've been recommended www.patient.co.uk and www.patient slikeme.com. My advice is, approach with caution.

Palliative and hospice care

Both of us have been blessed with good doctors and carers, who have guided us through the progress of our MND. Their worth far outweighs websites and they would always be my first source of advice. At some time one has to come to terms with one's utter dependence and impending death. And then there are also resources to help. In the

UK and RSA we are fortunate to have access to palliative nursing and hospice care, for example: Macmillan Cancer Care – www.macmillan.org.uk – which is not in fact confined to cancer care, and w ww.helpthehospices.org.uk. Since you might want to find your local hospice, you can search for that on line. But unsurprisingly one does need a doctor's referral. local hospice, you can search for that on line. But unsurprisingly one does need a doctor's referral.

Bereavement

And when the family have to cope with their loss, there are also groups to help. The Christian charity, Care for the Family, provides a useful list under 'Living with Loss': www.careforthefamily.org .uk.

Carers' support

For the support of carers, there are www.carers uk.org and www.nhs.uk/carersdirect. If you're faced with the bureaucracy of state support, for example claiming benefits, and www.nhs.uk/carersdirect. If you're faced with thebureaucracy of state support, for example claiming benefits, the Citizens' Advice Bureau and the Dial UK network (www.dialuk.info) are good resources. Another good UK site is the Princess Royal Trust for Carers (www.carers.org).

Campaigning groups

The major alliance of organizations opposed to euthanasia and assisted suicide is Care Not Killing – www.carenotkilling.org.uk. I think this is the best source of information and articles. Although it's not a specifically Christian alliance, many of the organizations involved are, not unexpectedly, faith-based. Organizations which campaign especially to protect the rights organizations involved are, not unexpectedly, faith-based. Organizations which campaign especially to protect the rights of the disabled include Not Dead Yet (www.notdeadyetuk.org) and No Less Human (www.spuc.org.uk/about/no-lesshuman).

The Church

Above all, your local church should provide you with the practical, emotional and spiritual support you need. That is its vocation and the test of its love: "'...And when did we see you sick or in prison and visit you?' And the King will answer them, 'Truly, I say to you, as you did it to one of the least of these my brothers, you did it to me'" (Matthew 25:39–s40). There are no more imprisoning sicknesses than those which lead to disability and death. This is Jesus' challenge to his Church. And for both of us our Christian communities have passed the test, perhaps not perfectly, but we are continually thankful to God for their love.

Back Cover Material

Jozanne Moss, in South Africa, and Michael Wenham in Britain, have only met by email. Both struggle daily with the condition known as Motor Neurone (or Lou Gehrig's) Disease, a progressive and ultimately fatal condition. Both are married to remarkable people who support and care for them.

Through Jozanne's story they address the myth that God is only responsible for the good bits in life. Michael explains: "God has brought us together with the same illness and the same goal: to encourage and inspire others with the life God has purposed for us."

Their story is wonderfully uplifting, made radiant by the faith of the two authors. Michael's own story is told in his book *My Donkeybody.*

"The writers' frank first-hand style tells it as it is ... Their faith helps them make sense of the chaos of living. Healthcare professionals should read this."

– **Baroness Professor Ilora Finlay,** patron of the MND Association

Jozanne and Michael offer a deep, careful and rich engagement with the Bible in the midst of the daily reality of terminal illness. They tackle hugely important issues with honesty and vulnerability."

– **Revd Nicky Gumbel,** Holy Trinity Brompton

"This book is a triumph. It is important and beautiful and incredible. And for me, personally, a deeply reflective journey."

– **Louise Halling** (who has Muscular Dystrophy) Sydney, Australia

Made in the USA
Monee, IL
05 November 2026

67808604R00149